Mind Over Fatter

A 30-Day Overhaul of the Mindset that has Sabotaged Your Fitness and Weight-loss Success

Mind Over Fatter

A 30-Day Overhaul of the Mindset that has Sabotaged Your Fitness and Weight-loss Success

By Gina Paolino
—A.M.P.F.T. Certified
 Personal Trainer
 with Honors
—B.A. Psychology,
 University of Massachusetts
 at Lowell
—Owner of Home Bodies
 in-home fitness training
 and consulting

Copyright © 2005 by Gina Paolino.
Cover artwork copyright © 2005 by Jeffrey Paulhus.

Cover design by Ed Goss.

All rights reserved, including the right of reproduction in whole or in part, in any form or by any means, electronic or mechanical, including photocopying, recording, or by any information or retrieval system, without the prior written permission of the author, except in the case of brief quotations embodied in magazines, newspapers or broadcasts.

Printed in the United States of America by King Printing.

The author of this book intends for this publication to provide accurate information. It is sold with the understanding that it is meant to complement, not be a substitute for, professional medical, rehabilitative, psychological, and/or health and fitness services.

ISBN:

First Printing: November 2004

Photo credits:
All photos are of Gina Paolino, courtesy of Bryan Paulhus and Hard Nock's Gym in Amesbury, MA.

This book is dedicated to Mom, Dad, Gram, Nana and Bryan. Thank you for being loving and supportive through my schooling and as I've worked to build my business.

Also to George and Debi, my gymnastics coaches for 7 years. They treat their gymnasts like one of the family. They've helped me develop character and toughness that take you very far in life.

And finally to Magdita, the one who inspired me to start my business.

This System is backed by my 100% cash back, no-questions-asked Lifetime Guarantee.

If you follow this program in its entirety and fail to achieve the results promised, please feel free to take advantage of my money-back Lifetime Guarantee.

Furthermore, if you are not satisfied with the System and do not feel you have received fair value for your money, please feel free to take advantage of my Lifetime Guarantee.

Contents

Part I. Greetings

Part II. Metabolism Primer
The Fundamentals of Metabolism 22
Energy Balance 28
The 7 Keys to Raising Your Metabolism for Life 50

Part III. Prep Work
Strategy 1. No Fear!
    How to make a commitment to change 69
Strategy 2. Stop Procrastinating
    How to increase your productivity and decrease your stress level 80
Strategy 3. Talking "up"
    How to use positive self-talk to promote success 86
Strategy 4. You are the Feature Presentation
    How to visualize success 90
Strategy 5. Applying discipline and creating S.M.A.R.T. Goals
    How goal-mapping ensures your success 94
Strategy 6. Developing a plan of action
    How to organize your goals into daily, short-term, and long-term 101
Strategy 7. Fine-toothed comb
    How to be sure of success 105

Part IV. Taking the Plunge
Strategy 8. What's Up Doc?
    Consulting with your Physician 112
Strategy 9. It's a Breeze
    How to easily implement your action plan 115
Strategy 10. I'm Obsessed
    How to make your goals a positive obsession 122
Strategy 11. A spoonful of sugar
    How to create a supportive exercise atmosphere 130
Strategy 12. Decisions, decisions
    Choosing your health and fitness resources 134

Part V. The Daily Grind
Strategy 13. If you fail to plan, you plan to fail
    How to rehearse for success 145
Strategy 14. Hocus Focus
    How to concentrate during exercise and eating to maximize results 148
Strategy 15. Short-Term Sacrifice –
Food Cravings and Exercise Avoidance
    How to overcome the need for instant gratification that will sabotage your success 153
Strategy 16. Really *Needing* it
    How to make success a necessity in your life 168

Strategy 17. Just do *something*
How exercise action and mini-workouts yield results   172
Strategy 18. Time on your side
How to make the time to be a regular exerciser   177
Strategy 19. Do it right or don't do it at all
Strict form makes all the difference   187
Strategy 20. Better safe than sorry
How to exercise to get healthy, not to get injured   191
Strategy 21. 48-hour rule: Leave that muscle alone!
How rest allows you to progress even faster   200
Strategy 22. The stronger, the better
How to use strength and performance as a results indicator   204
Strategy 23. Just right
Choosing the right resistance   211
Strategy 24. Racking up those miles
How cardiovascular work fits into the picture   219

Part VI. Anti-Stagnant
Strategy 25. Time to work out *again*?
Avoid getting bored with exercise   232
Strategy 26. Surprise, surprise!
Keep mixing things up   237
Strategy 27. Strain to Gain
How to push through your exercise comfort zone   240
Strategy 28. Handle with care.
How to treat your body right   247
Strategy 29. Sit down already!
Why rest is crucial to achieving the body you want   252
Strategy 30. Congratulate yourself!
How to completely enjoy and appreciate all that you've accomplished   258

Part VII. Reference
Reference A. "The 10 Tricks You Need to Know to Eat Right, one person at a time"   262
Reference B. Nutrition Guidelines
    General Nutrition Guidelines   268
    The 80/20 Rule and Eating in Moderation   272
    Artificial Sweeteners   276
    Alcohol   281
    Eating Out the Healthy Way   283
    Fast-Food on a Diet   287
Reference C. "Just How Much Time is Required to Experience the Benefits of Exercise?"   289
    Fit with Four   291
    "Progressive Resistance Cycle Training"
    A systematic, scientific approach to your exercise routine   306
Reference D. Body Types and Training Suggestions   312
Reference E. Sources of Information on Diet and Training   321
Notes and Index   323

I. Greetings

Welcome! Before we get started, I'd like to thank you for putting your trust in me by purchasing this System. I want to assure you that I've spent a great deal of time and energy researching and testing the information in this book and I have 100% confidence that it works. Before we get any further, though, I'm going to tell you a little bit about me.

My name is Gina Paolino, and I'm the owner of Home Bodies in-home fitness training. My business provides fitness training services, health and fitness coaching and consulting, and personalized exercise and nutrition plans. I also write original health and fitness articles, a monthly Newsletter, and health and fitness books like this one. You can find all these things and more at my company's website, www.homeexercisecoach.com. I provide most of my services and programs in-home. I also work with clients at the Seacoast Family YMCA in Portsmouth, New Hampshire and at Hard Nock's Gym in Amesbury, Massachusetts.

I am nationally certified fitness trainer, and have over eight years of experience in the health and fitness industry. I competed in gymnastics for ten years and have been a gymnastics coach for eight years. I also have a bachelor's degree in psychology and business. One of my greatest passions is psychology and its application in behavioral change. In fact, fitness, nutrition, and psychology are all passions of mine and I spend a great deal of time researching these topics. I like to go beyond theory by testing the techniques I learn on people in the real world. My health and fitness programs consist of a blend of applications that come from the fields of biology, exercise physiology, nutrition, and psychology. All of my programs are geared toward helping people develop and maintain a healthy, fit body. My ultimate goal is for every one of my customers and clients to be healthy, in shape, and full of energy. Last, but certainly not least, I want them to look great too.

This System will lead you step-by-step in uncovering your own sources of internal motivation for exercising and eating better. You'll also learn how you can turn the forces in your environment into sources of external motivation. This System will serve as a guide in helping you set up your own personalized health and fitness program. If you feel like you've tried everything to lose weight and get in shape and failed at each one, this System is exactly what you need because nothing is left to chance. This System covers all bases, including the physiology of what works and what doesn't, mental and psychological aspects of diet and training, and the planning, implementation, and adaptation of your program over time.

This System is the only book I've seen that ties *all* the important issues together and explains them in everyday language. I feel it's important for you to understand *why* these techniques work because it's motivating to understand the purpose behind the work you'll need to do to get in shape. I'm *not* going to tell you what to do or what not to do, but I *am* going to educate you so that you can make your own decisions.

The purpose of this System is to help you make positive, lasting changes in your life. Specifically, my goal is for you to enjoy a boost in your physical and mental health, your fitness level, and, as a result of all that, your appearance. If you decide to follow the Strategies outlined here, you will find that many aspects of your life begin to improve. It is not especially difficult to work through the Strategies in this program, but it *will* require a solid commitment from you. You won't need "willpower" to make the changes I ask – you simply need to be capable of making a commitment and following instructions, and you'll need to have patience and faith during the process. You can be assured that many before you have applied the Strategies in my System and have incredible results to show for it. This is the first time my System has been available in a comprehensive form – up until now I've been educating my clients through my Newsletter, my articles, and our one-on-one sessions. Now that I've had plenty of time to test my ideas, I feel an obligation to reach more people with this life-changing information. This System is designed to be a motivational book, a behavior modification program, and a health and fitness resource that I hope will be helpful to you and your loved ones for years and years to come.

As you prepare to start using this System, realize that there's no reason to feel intimidated. Everything that I require as part of the program is well within the capabilities of everyday people – don't worry, you are not going to be expected to run a marathon or deadlift 200 pounds. Those feats of stamina and strength, although impressive, are certainly not requirements for being a fit and healthy person. The only challenge I'll pose to you is in asking you to commit yourself to this process, as it *will* require work on your part. As the owner of a personal training business, I would love to be able to sell you a magic pill that could instantly improve your health, your fitness, and your overall well-being. Believe me, it would make everything easier for both of us! Since nothing like that exists, I will offer you the next best thing: A science-based program that addresses physical, emotional, and psychological needs, along with my promise and personal guarantee that it works.

First, though, I have one request for you: I prefer that you don't start dabbling in any of the Strategies you are about to learn if you're not willing to stick with it for 30 days. Whether it's one Strategy or all thirty that you'd like to try at the outset, your chances of making a permanent change are dramatically reduced if you don't commit to giving it an honest try for at least a month's time. If you go through this program just trying things halfheartedly, you won't be able to see the value in the Strategies and they will lose their power.

For the sake of clarification, I want you to know that I have no problem with you reading through this System and deciding that you're not ready to make any change at this time. The moment when you feel ready is your call – no one will be able to force you. Regardless of whether you're ready to give one Strategy a go or you'd like to try the 30-day program in its entirety, I would like you to mark off the 30 days on your calendar during which you will maintain your commitment to the Strategies.

To understand the reasoning behind this request, you need a little more background on where I'm coming from. The reason I became a fitness trainer who also writes about health, fitness, and motivation is that I want to spread the life-enhancing information I have to as many people as possible. I want to be of service for things that *really* make a difference for people. If you pass off my System as "just another weight-loss gimmick that doesn't work" you will detract from my mission, which is to deliver sound, expert advice to as many people as possible. When you apply my System the way it's designed, you'll be so successful that I know you'll help me get the message out by spreading the word to others wanting help with their weight, health, appearance, and quality of life. So I beg you to give 100% in your attempt to apply the information contained in this System.

If you don't feel ready at this point in your life to take a serious gander at the material, just put the program aside and come back to it later on when you're so fed up that you're not only *willing* but actually *eager* to make a change. Or, consider passing my System along to someone who seems ready today to work on his health and fitness. Who knows – if he does well using this System, you might be inspired to try too!

This 30-day program is about doing *something* nearly every day, rather than doing an extreme amount on any given day. This program *isn't* a quick fix, but it *will* serve you well for the rest of your life if you continue to follow the principles.

Before you start working this System, keep in mind that I am requesting a 30-day commitment on your part – if you don't think maintaining the changes is worth it or you don't look and feel better, you can always go back to your old ways. I'm asking just 30 days during which you'll commit to giving it an honest try. Most people find, once they get over the first 30-day hump, that exercise and eating better is *definitely* worth it. I'd like for you to think of this as a process of breaking an "addiction" to an unhealthy lifestyle or an unhealthy behavior. While you are in the midst of an unhealthy lifestyle, it is all you know. If you can break free from that situation and turn to look at your former lifestyle from the outside in, most likely you will realize that you don't ever want to go back there again. As an added bonus, your new, healthier ways of living will have become habits after the first 3-4 weeks – the changes will be much, much easier to stick to at that point.

When you look at it that way, it's no wonder why certain people seem to hit the ground running (literally!) when they start exercising and eating better. You've seen their profiles in the magazines – the ones who used to eat fast-food three times a day and considered a workout to be actually walking inside versus using the drive-thru – and then they became a poster-child for the local gym and the natural foods store. Along the way, they lost ten inches off their gut and gained a ton of energy and confidence. These people aren't any "better" than you – it's just that once they "flipped the switch" they really didn't have the *option* to go back because they realized all the good feelings they had been missing out on while they were too busy neglecting their bodies. See, when you look at exercise and eating well as a means to *gain more good feelings* rather than as a way to *lose fun and happiness*, you'll start looking at junk food and sedentary living in a different light. Sure, they can be short-term pleasures at times, but they're always a source of pain in the end. Upon reaching that realization, the choice of what to do becomes automatic.

Okay, so if you're with me in thinking that this health and fitness stuff might be worth it, what to do? If you're like most Americans you want everything *now*, and if you could have it *yesterday* you would take that too. Needless to say, patience isn't exactly a strong suit for most of us. That impatience is what sparks the fire that fuels the $45-billion U.S. weight-loss industry.

There are some products out there that claim they can help you lose 10 pounds in three days, or other impressive feats. Even if these claims *are* true (and everyone knows they almost always *are not,* or else the entire weight-loss industry would be turned on it's head), who's to say that you'll keep the weight off, or that you won't have to keep buying and using the product forever to continue enjoying the benefit?

The beauty of a behavior and lifestyle modification program like this one is that the knowledge and power you gain learning and applying the System can serve you over and over if needed, at no additional cost beyond the time you put into the process. This isn't a pill or a gym membership that you have to keep paying for over and over, lest you fall back into being out-of-shape. And, although this System is more time-intensive than popping a pill, it's definitely time well spent. Following the program will result in a healthier, happier, and more productive life. You'll also become more self-sufficient and intrinsically motivated as you work this System, since you'll begin to reap the rewards that are simply natural consequences of living healthfully. In addition to tapping sources of internal motivation, you'll learn how to use external motivators to your advantage to reinforce the behaviors that will make your life better. Perhaps most importantly, you will stop being a victim of the forces in your environment that make it harder by the year to stay on top of your health, your fitness, and your weight.

Even though my program is simple to follow, if you don't approach the steps systematically it'll be easy to get distracted or feel overwhelmed. My System, when followed sequentially, is a *foolproof* method for putting the necessary cognitive and behavioral changes for getting fit and losing fat into action. It's extremely powerful and worth more than its weight in gold when applied correctly. What you hold in your hands is powerful enough to finally release you from the vicious cycle of unhealthy habits that sabotage your success and your ability to experience complete happiness.

If you looked through the Contents, you might have noticed that the System includes 30 Strategies, each focusing on one key concept. If you have a history of rushing into things full-force and quitting them just as suddenly, your best bet is to make a 30-day commitment to read and focus on one Strategy a day. This will give you the chance to establish a rock-solid foundation in the Strategies. Hopefully, that process will inspire and motivate you so that you will be ready to make the commitment to actually apply the material – and applying the material is the *only* way that you'll get to enjoy all the positive changes that will come into your life when you're living healthfully. Once you've had the opportunity to familiarize yourself with the Strategies (your first 30-day commitment), you can start a new 30-day commitment – one that will involve working the assignments in addition to actually living the healthy habits.

Now, I realize that some of you will want to start living the healthy habits immediately. If you are determined to start your healthy lifestyle as soon as possible, you will need to skim the entire program and study the Reference section closely so that you can formulate your health and fitness goals that will become the cornerstone of your program. Once you have given yourself an overview of the information, be sure to follow the System in order and complete all of the assignments while you are in the midst of your 30-day healthier-living commitment. The Strategies in this program appear in the order they will be needed. Therefore, if you wish to take the "fast track" and keep up with reading one Strategy a day, you should be able to read and study the Strategies during the same 30-day time period that you are actually applying the program.

If, upon flipping through the System, it looks like it will be time-consuming, you're not imagining things – this certainly isn't an overnight solution. Moreover, I'm not expecting everyone to follow every Strategy or try everything that's included in this book. However, I *am* assuming that you are reading this right now because you're serious about improving your health and fitness. I have no interest in publishing a "fluff" book that really doesn't offer much in the way of helpful information for an intelligent person. Besides, once you're rolling, the actual program doesn't take very much time. Going through the Strategies and assignments at the outset is the part that's going to be a little more time-intensive. However, the time you spend up-front is what will enable you to set up your program to run as smoothly and efficiently as possible. In the end, you will come out ahead if you take the time to focus on this project for a little while. You can think of it as a crash course in making these important changes in your life – it will be intense for a little while, but it will be over soon and then you'll have your program up and running as smooth as can be. If you follow the instructions as laid out in this System, your actual workout routine will never have to take more than a few hours per week. Remember, everything new can be overwhelming at first, but it won't feel that way for long.

<u>If you already follow a fairly healthy lifestyle and are just looking to learn more, pick and choose the Strategies you'd like to follow and keep the "7 Keys" and Reference sections in mind for times when you'd like a refresher in the fundamental topics of health and fitness.</u> Also, keep your eyes peeled for my upcoming titles that

will delve more extensively into advanced health and fitness topics.

I know that some of you are reading this as one of my Home Bodies, Hard Nock's Gym, or Seacoast Family YMCA clients. You will surely recognize some of the ideas presented in this System. Hopefully, you will enjoy this book as a health and fitness resource and it will help supplement your appointments with me. I thank all of you from the bottom of my heart for your trust, friendship, continuing support of my business, and referrals. I wish the absolute best for you and your loved ones.

I'd like to give special thanks to new clients in 2004 who also happen to be really great people: Susan Anderson, Nancy Angell, Greg Beadle, Courtney Bernier, Dawn Blanchard, Jeff Brown, Judy Chretian, Dee Cote, Dawn Cundy, Barbara Devincenzo, Ingrid Dicenzo, Fenn Duncan, Chris Ferreira, Ellen Hazo, Kathi Jaibur, Jean Lambert, Tiffany Landsperger, Bill McDill, Loretta Meleedy, Jim Miller, Loretta Moseley, Brian Moses, Janet Moses, Lynn Noyes, Kelly Page, Jeffrey Paolino, Diane Pendergast, Tom Pendergast, Sabina Petersen, Susan Reaney, Christine Rivers, Ann Salmon, Heather Siegel, Soni Soulagnet, Magdalena Suarez-Shannon, Francine Vozzella, Donna Winner, and Jim Winner. I'd also like to give special thanks to Dave Nock, owner of Hard Nock's Gym in Amesbury, MA.

II. Metabolism Primer

The Fundamentals of Metabolism

Understanding metabolism is critical if you're going to take control of your health, your weight, your fitness, and your energy level. What is metabolism anyway? Even though "metabolism" is a buzzword today, most people only have a vague idea of what it means, although they *do* know that theirs seems to have slowed down lately! I'll give you a quick explanation of what metabolism is, what affects it, and what you can do to increase yours right away.

In simple terms, metabolism is the rate at which your body burns fuel to sustain life and all of the processes that take place in your body. The main factors that affect metabolism are activity level, eating habits, muscle tissue, and genetics.

The relationship between metabolism and activity level is pretty straightforward – the more active you are, the more calories you burn. Daily living and exercise combine to form your activity level.

Eating habits is another factor that can have a big impact on your metabolism. *How often you eat* and *what you eat* are equally important because both directly affect your blood sugar and energy levels. Unstable blood sugar causes the metabolism to slow down as a means to conserve energy. That's why skipping breakfast (or any meal for that matter) is the worst thing you can do for your metabolism.

Muscle development has a huge effect on your metabolism, and building and conditioning your muscles represents your biggest opportunity to increase your metabolic rate. The more muscle tissue you have, the higher your metabolism will be. Having sufficient muscle mass is a prerequisite to having a youthful, toned body. Also, when you have a good amount of muscle mass you'll find it much easier to manage your weight. Muscle burns calories, and the more you have the better! Not only does exercising the muscles burn lots of calories, maintaining more muscle on your body also means you burn more calories all day, every day – even while you're sleeping! Therefore, embarking on a resistance-training program is a no-brainer for dieters. How many people have you heard say their metabolism has changed as they've aged? The main reason these people start to put on weight more easily is that they've experienced a loss of muscle mass over the years. You lose muscle and body tone due to a lack of physical exercise and unstable blood sugar – contrary to the common misconception that muscle loss is simply a natural part of aging. More accurately, muscle loss is just a "natural part" of not exercising your muscles on a consistent basis.

There is also a genetic component to metabolism. Some people have faster metabolisms than average, while others tend to have slower ones. Still, no matter where you fall within the genetic variation, you can always increase your metabolism if you use the right approach.

Now that you have a general overview of metabolism and what affects it, I'm going to reveal the two most powerful things you can do to increase your metabolism:

1. Develop and condition your muscle tissue (usually, although not necessarily, by increasing the size of your muscles) with progressive resistance training.

2. Stabilize your blood sugar level and energy balance throughout the day. Due to hormonal implications in the body, keeping your energy intake steady during the day promotes fat loss and helps prevent additional fat storage. This can be accomplished by eating small meals every few hours, each containing a moderate amount of carbohydrate, protein, and fat.

Taking control of your metabolism is actually pretty easy if you know what to do, and you *don't* need to exercise more than a few days per week to do it. Besides the two techniques I've already introduced for increasing metabolism, I'm going to discuss five more that will help in your quest to raise your metabolism for life. Altogether, these tips make up the "7 Keys" to raising metabolism, which I will detail later in this section of the book

Before we go any further, though, I would like to differentiate between a few terms I will be using throughout this book. The word "diet" technically refers to a person's typical way of eating (it doesn't necessarily refer to a weight-loss plan). So, someone who habitually overeats has a "high-calorie diet," while someone who eats less in order to lose weight has a "low-calorie diet." Throughout this book, I will use the term "diet" in this technical or dictionary-definition sense, which is to describe various ways of eating, whether or not that way of eating is likely to result in a change in weight.

However, <u>in this book I'm going to take the liberty to use the term "dieting" to mean what the general public perceives it to mean – the process of eating in a certain way to promote weight loss. A "dieter," then, will be a person who is trying to eat in a certain way</u>

to promote weight loss.

If you're looking to shed pounds, a common approach is to start by restricting your calories, meaning to restrict your energy intake from food. In other words, you'll be dieting by reducing or even eliminating consumption of certain *types* of food (such as following a low-carb or low-fat plan), or by cutting back on the *amount* of food you eat by watching portion sizes and/or watching what you eat between meals.

Everyone requires a certain number of calories per day to maintain bodyweight. By dieting, the goal is to consume fewer calories than you burn each day, otherwise known as "running a calorie deficit." The total number of calories you burn per day is your maintenance calorie level. By definition, if you eat at your maintenance calorie level your weight won't change. Your maintenance calorie level depends on your metabolism, which in turn depends on the four factors I discussed above: activity level, eating habits, muscle tissue, and genetics. Sometimes your maintenance calorie level will be a range rather than an exact number. If you have a range for your maintenance calorie level, you have to eat outside of that range in order to affect a change in your weight. For example, you might maintain your weight on anything from 2000-2400 calories per day, meaning that you'd have to eat less than 2000 on a regular basis to lose weight, or more than 2400 on a regular basis to gain weight.

If you reduce your calorie intake to below maintenance, and therefore are running a calorie deficit, by definition you will lose weight. And, if you *continue* to run a calorie deficit by consuming less than you burn day after day, you will *continue* to lose weight. As many of us know, this is easier said than done. More often than not, when you try to diet by cutting calories it doesn't last very long because you get sick of feeling moody, hungry, and tired. Sometimes, the problem is simply a matter of feeling deprived – you don't like missing out on all the things you used to eat.

Enduring physical and psychological discomfort is not the only hard part of dieting, however. The other problem with plain-old calorie restriction is that, as you lose weight, you will need to eat fewer and fewer calories as time goes on if you want to continue to lose. There are two reasons for this. The first is that a smaller body requires fewer calories. The second is that your metabolism will begin to slow in response to a reduced calorie intake. When less energy is available, your body perceives the calorie shortage as a threat to survival and will begin to take drastic measures to conserve energy. These changes include a lowered body temperature, reduced heart rate, general lethargy, increase in bodyfat, decrease in lean tissue, and a change in hormonal levels that results in the functioning of some of the body systems slowing down – most notably the "nonessential" systems.

One such system is the one responsible for protein synthesis in the muscles. This body system, known as the "metabolic system," is responsible for building and maintaining muscle mass. Remember how I said that muscle burns calories? That is exactly what your body *doesn't* need when it feels threatened by a low calorie intake. Your body can "kill two birds with one stone" by breaking down muscle tissue when it wants to conserve energy. When muscle tissue is broken down into amino acids and burned for fuel, it provides a source of calories for the body, and at the same time your body eliminates the need to feed that muscle extra calories in the future. Of course, that's bad news for the dieter who wants to burn all the extra calories he can.

The immune system is another "nonessential" system that starts to slow down in response to a low calorie intake. Your body won't allocate as much energy toward fighting off illness when it's trying to fight for survival from a perceived threat of starvation. When the body feels that it's at risk for starving to death, everything becomes secondary to the need to obtain more food.

The reproductive system is the third "nonessential" system that starts shutting down when you're not eating many calories. Libido drops, again, because the body's main concern is to prevent itself from starving to death. Reproduction, which of course is related to libido, takes a secondary role when there's a perceived threat of starvation (this is one reason why women may stop menstruating and men sometimes become impotent if they cut calories too hard or lose most of their bodyfat). The loss of libido makes sense on another level too – if survival is already being threatened, the last thing you need is to reproduce, because that means you'll have even more people around to compete for the scarce resources!

Your body wants one thing when it's deprived of calories, and that's to find food and eat it, fast! This explains why many dieters become obsessed with food – and sometimes that doesn't ever go away, even when a dieter goes off his diet and begins to eat more calories, and even when his bodyfat stores are plentiful.

With all the negative implications of low-calorie diets, it seems that there has to be a better solution for weight loss! Luckily, there is. You have another option to lose weight besides cutting calories, because the other side of your energy (or calorie) balance – the number of calories you burn per day – isn't set in stone. *If you start burning more calories than you used to, you will be able to keep eating the same amount of food, or in some cases even more food than you had been eating, and lose weight at the same time.* Losing weight while eating a "normal" amount of food is an easier and healthier way to diet, both from a physical and a psychological standpoint. You can increase the number of calories you burn per day by following the "7 Keys to Raising Your Metabolism for Life" which I will describe shortly.

One rule of thumb to keep in mind is that calorie burn increases when daily activity goes up. One way to increase daily activity is through exercise. Many people who want to lose weight will perform moderate-pace cardiovascular exercise (such as brisk walking or easy jogging) because they know that it burns calories. "Burning" calories is really just another way of saying that you've raised your maintenance calorie level. When you raise your maintenance calorie level but don't eat any more to compensate, you'll lose weight.

For example, if you have been eating about 2000 calories per day while maintaining your weight and would like to lose weight, you have a couple of choices. One option is to start eating fewer calories. If you choose this option, you might cut out 500 calories and eat just 1500 per day.

Creating an energy deficit

			Eat	Burn		
			x	x		
0	500	1000	1500	2000	2500	calories/day

Another option for weight loss is to continue eating the same amount but increase your activity level during the day, whether you do that at work, at play, through exercise, or all of the above. When you become more active, your daily calorie needs go up. Using the current example, taking the extra activity into account your maintenance calorie level is now higher than 2000 per day – it might go up to 2500 when you begin adding more activity into your day. This means, if you continue to eat just 2000 calories, you will lose weight.

Creating an energy deficit

				Eat	Burn	
				x	x	
0	500	1000	1500	2000	2500	calories/day

You might be wondering why you couldn't eat less *and* move more in order to lose weight even faster. This will work to a point, but you need to understand that your best bet for fat loss is to maintain the optimal calorie deficit – not too small, but not too large either. This concept is known as "energy balance" and you can read about it on the next page.

Energy Balance

How large should your calorie deficit be? In other words, by how much should you be looking to "undereat" or "overburn" to lose the greatest amount of fat and the least amount of muscle, and at the same time remain healthy and energetic? These questions refer to the concept of energy balance. Calories are the way in which we measure the energy provided by food. Energy balance in the context of human metabolism refers to calories-in versus calories-out.

A 150-pound woman will burn roughly 1500 calories just to maintain her body weight before typical daily activity is taken into account. "Typical daily activity" refers to any movement beyond simply resting in bed. The 1500 calories is her basal metabolic rate (BMR). If the woman works full-time, walks her dog, and does a few errands during the day, she has a moderate level of daily activity, and probably burns another 500 calories on top of her BMR. This makes her daily calorie burn before exercise 2000 calories. If she also performs cardiovascular exercise at a moderate-pace for 30 minutes, she might burn another 200 calories, and if she completes a 30-minute resistance training program she might burn an additional 200 calories. After everything has been taken into consideration, during a day like this she burns around 2400 calories.

Calories Burned

			Bed Only	w/ Daily Life	w/ Weights and Cardio	
			X	X	X	
0	500	1000	1500	2000	2500	calories/day

The human body is capable of burning about 0.5-2.0 pounds of bodyfat per week as an energy source (to supply calories to cover the calorie deficit). The exact ceiling for what's possible in terms of bodyfat loss depends on a person's size, activity level, and individual metabolism. In other words, larger people and more active people generally are able to lose fat faster than smaller people and less active people. However, each person has her own metabolic rate, which means there is individual variation in how fast a person can lose bodyfat. Generally, if you weigh less than 170 pounds you won't be able to lose in the upper range of 1.5-2.0 pounds of bodyfat per week, at least not on a regular basis. The reason is that the amount of bodyfat you can lose in a day is actually based on percentage of total body weight. This makes sense if you think about it, because a 5-pound weight loss on a 120-pound frame is comparable to a 10-pound weight loss on a 240-pound frame.

You need to burn about 3500 calories without replacing them with calories from food in order to burn off one pound of bodyfat. Each pound of fat you burn supplies 3500 calories to the body to cover your calorie deficit. If you'd like to shoot for the respectable goal of losing one pound of bodyfat in a week, you'll need to burn an average of 500 calories per day beyond the number you consume, and you'll need to do that for seven days (500 calories x 7 days = 3500 calories, or one pound of fat).

You may be wondering why you can sometimes lose a pound (or three) *in a day* when you weigh yourself on the scale. This type of fluctuation in bodyweight is due to a change in water weight, and water weight can come on and off quickly. All you have to do to "gain" a pound is drink a 16-ounce bottle of water! A person's weight on the scale can vary within a 10-pound range in some cases, even when there is no change in the amount of muscle or bodyfat he's carrying. The difference in weight on the scale is due to the amount of water and carbohydrate being stored in the body. Each gram of carbohydrate stored in the body holds about 3 grams of water along with it, which can add up fast because your muscles have the ability to store 500-1300 grams of carbs or more, depending on the amount of lean body mass you carry and the conditioning of your muscles (weight-training increases your body's ability to store carbs in the muscles). According to the scale, you might lose five pounds or more the first week of a diet because there is a loss of water weight associated with running the calorie deficit that is necessary for fat loss (Unless you have been eating almost nothing and exercising for hours and hours every day, you surely haven't created a calorie deficit to the tune of 17,500 calories in just seven days! That's what it would take to lose five pounds of actual bodyfat). After that initial reduction in water weight, however, each pound lost on the scale when you monitor your weight on a weekly basis should represent an actual loss of bodyfat. Of course, this is assuming you're not dieting too hard and you're doing your resistance training. If you *are* dieting too hard or you're *not* doing resistance training, your weight loss most likely will be from a combination of muscle loss and fat loss.

Many of the weight-loss products out there today are designed to reduce water weight, which is only a temporary change. However, this change on the scale happens quickly and is a relatively painless occurrence for the dieter, which equates to the perfect short-term solution for the average person who wants results *now*! Of course, in the long run nothing has happened at all. But people still buy into this stuff to the tune of $45-billion a year. By the same token, you can overeat for a day and see the scale climb 5 pounds or more, but that represents just a temporary gain in water weight. True fat gain and fat loss is a much slower process, and to gain a pound of bodyfat you'd have to eat 3500 calories *beyond your maintenance level* (putting you up above 5500 calories consumed in a single day). Can it be done? Sure. Will most people be able to overeat by that much, even if they tried? No.

Let's go back to our example of the 150-pound woman with a theoretical maintenance calorie level before exercise of 2000 calories per day. She has several choices if she wants to run a calorie deficit in order to lose bodyfat. If she didn't do any cardio on one particular day but completed a resistance training routine (or vice-versa, since we estimated that each would burn 200 calories), she would burn 2200 calories that day. This means she needs to eat 1700 to run a deficit of 500 calories for the day and be on track to lose one pound of bodyfat per week. When you run a calorie deficit, there is a discrepancy between the number of calories you consume and the number of calories you burn. The calories you burn above and beyond your food intake to create your calorie deficit have to come from somewhere (no, it's not like the national budget deficit!), and it turns out that, as long as you exercise, they usually come from your bodyfat as it's burned for energy.

500-calories' worth of fat loss

				Eat	Burn	
				x	x	
0	500	1000	1500	2000	2500	calories/day

If the woman does both cardio and resistance training, she burns 2400 calories (2000 before exercise, 200 for cardio and 200 for resistance training), and therefore needs to eat 1900 calories in order to create a 500-calorie deficit.

500-calories' worth of fat loss

				Eat	Burn	
				x	x	
0	500	1000	1500	2000	2500	calories/day

What happens if she does resistance training plus 60 minutes of cardio and only eats 1000 calories? If she does 60 minutes of cardio rather than the 30 minutes we've been using as an example, her total daily calorie burn is 2600, up from 2400 (assuming that each 30 minutes of cardio burns 200 calories). If she eats only 1000 calories that day, she will be running a 1600-calorie deficit. Unfortunately, not all of the calories making up that deficit will come from bodyfat being burned for energy. In fact, if she creates a 1600-calorie deficit for more than a day or two, most of the necessary calories will be provided by lean tissue being burned for energy, which will cause her metabolism to slow down. Having a slower metabolism means that she burns fewer calories tomorrow, even if she maintains the same activity level (If she lowers her calories that drastically just for a day or two, she won't be at risk for slowing her metabolism – but all that will happen is she'll start using up her stored muscle glycogen as an energy source. Still, she won't be burning much, if any, more bodyfat than she would have burned just by sticking to the recommended 500-calorie deficit).

If she depletes her muscle glycogen by eating a very-low-calorie diet and exercising vigorously a few days in a row, she will lose several pounds of water weight and perhaps 1750 calories' worth, or a half-pound, of bodyfat (which is about the same amount she would have lost just sticking to the 500-calorie deficit). However, the depletion of muscle glycogen will leave her weak and tired, and her exercise performance and motivation will take a nosedive. The crash dieting also sets her up to break her diet big-time when the hunger and appetite increase due to the crash diet starts to kick in.

The situation I've described here is known as yo-yo dieting, and it's not pretty. Most people will end up breaking such a severe diet because the hunger and cravings they are almost sure to experience prove to be too difficult to endure. Let's assume, though, that this person maintains her crash diet for an entire week. Here's what her energy balance looks like on a daily basis:

500-calories' worth of fat loss, 1100-calories' worth of muscle loss and glycogen/water loss = a 1600-calorie deficit

		Eat			Burn	
		x			x	
0	500	1000	1500	2000	2500	calories/day

In general, the human body is not physiologically capable of losing nearly a half-pound of fat in a single day. That means the person who runs a 1600-calorie deficit every day will lose some fat *but more lean tissue*, and her body will in turn adjust its metabolism downward in order to conserve energy. This happens due to the body's survival mechanisms. Of course, a large calorie deficit for just one day won't result in a drastic change in metabolism, but if you string a few days together with a large calorie deficit, your metabolism will surely take a turn for the worse. And, it takes much longer for your metabolism to be brought back up to normal than it does for your metabolism to crash. The human body is designed to vigorously defend against fat loss, but the body accepts weight gain much more easily.

See, your body's primary concern is survival – even though you're dieting with the purpose of shedding excess bodyfat, your body's tendency is to fight fat loss tooth and nail, especially when it's not receiving a steady supply of calories. Your body's first step when faced with an energy crisis (a too-large calorie deficit) is to conserve fat stores, since they are the only thing that will keep you alive when food isn't readily available. When you restrict your food intake, your body has no way of knowing that you're not in the midst of a genuine famine. In fact, the newest diet pills and supplements in the works focus on tricking your body into thinking everything's okay and that plenty of calories are coming in. If these pills and supplements prove to be effective and become available, you will be able to diet without experiencing the metabolic slowdown that leads to a stall in your weight loss. It's important you understand that, during "famine" conditions, bodyfat is the most precious resource there is and it's the last thing your body is willing to let go. That's why it's important for you to eat on a regular basis while you're dieting, and also to avoid cutting calories too drastically. If you restrict calories too much, your body will simply fight back that much harder by conserving more energy. Heavy restriction of calories might work in the short-term to drop a few pounds, but it won't work in the long-term unless you're planning on starving yourself for the rest of your life – which isn't very realistic and definitely isn't healthy.

Due to the survival response, you'll find that the harder you cut calories, the more your body will intensify your hunger and appetite. Your body's first method of *defense* when there isn't enough food coming in is to slow the metabolism to conserve energy. Its primary methods of *attack* are to increase the secretion of stress hormones and intensify your hunger and appetite. The presence of stress hormones shuts down the nonessential systems in the body (a defense against a low calorie intake) and also stimulates you to stay alert in order to find food (an "attack" to rectify the low food supply), while the increased hunger and appetite further motivate you in your pursuit for nourishment (to energize your "attack" to find food). You become much more likely to crave calorie-dense foods (those high in fat and/or sugar) when you're not eating much, since those foods will provide the most calories to your body the quickest.

The survival mechanism is designed to motivate you to go find food and eat it as quickly as possible, because your body assumes that there is simply none around. The intense sensation of hunger you'll experience when you run a large calorie deficit makes it extremely difficult to continue to eat so little. In fact, the hunger you'll experience when you run a large calorie deficit makes it difficult to continue to maintain any calorie deficit at all, and it drives some dieters to break their diet on a binge. You have to realize that willpower has nothing to do with this. If you're like the majority of people, your body releases hormones that literally leave you powerless over what you will or will not eat. When you cut calories too hard or go for too long without eating, your body will fight you tooth and nail. When people don't understand this and they get upset with themselves for being "weak," their morale suffers and their confidence takes a hit. Once this has happened they start lacking the confidence that's necessary to succeed in weight loss. They start feeling like they deserve to look the way they do because they don't have any "willpower" when it comes to food. This notion becomes a downward spiral of negative thinking that quite often leads to self-sabotage. It literally traps people into a lifetime of health problems, low self-esteem, and unhappiness if no one shows them the way.

To make matters worse, when you cut calories too hard your body not only ramps up hunger to replace the calorie deficit you created while dieting, but it actually increases hunger above and beyond the magnitude of your deficit. The purpose? To encourage you to *overeat* in case there's another "famine" in the future. That way you'll have extra bodyfat in storage in case you're ever deprived of food again. Your body also primes itself to become *ultra-efficient at gaining weight* after a period of food restriction, again as part of the survival response. You can witness this phenomenon in action when you watch "yo-yo dieters" gain and lose weight over and over, more often than not gaining back more than they had lost with each episode. Even if yo-yo dieters manage to stay the same weight over time, after each episode of losing weight rapidly only to gain it back again they will be left with more bodyfat and less muscle. As you know, this combination is deadly for the metabolism. Bodyfat doesn't burn a significant number of extra calories, which means that overweight people don't necessarily burn more calories than thin people. It's the difference in *lean mass* that affects the number of calories burned per day, and you can't tell who has more lean mass simply by comparing what two people weigh on the scale. For instance, a lean person weighing 160 pounds at 10% bodyfat has 16 pounds of fat and 144 pounds of lean weight on his body, while an overweight person weighing 200 pounds at 30% bodyfat has 60 pounds of fat and just 140 pounds of lean weight on his body. The 160-pound person actually has 4 more pounds of lean weight on his body even though he's 40 pounds lighter – and, all other things being equal, has a higher metabolism as result.

It should be apparent to you by now that going on a severe diet is an exercise in futility. Even if, by some Herculean willpower, you manage to continue eating less and less over time to keep the weight off, you will eventually reach a point where your metabolism is so slow that you'll gain weight and bodyfat even on tiny amounts of food. That is the "reward" you'll get for all your efforts! However, there is a way around this problem: If you can be patient and are willing to settle for "only" 0.5-2.0 pounds of fat loss a week, you should be able to continue to lose excess bodyfat at that rate for months on end. With dieting, it really is true that "slow and steady wins the race."

See, the body is capable of burning bodyfat to provide fuel for all your daily activities, including exercise. There is a "ceiling" on how much bodyfat you can burn per day for energy, but the number of days your body will allow you to hit that ceiling is virtually unlimited. What is that ceiling? Well, if you undereat by approximately 500 calories per day (meaning that you're running a

500-calorie deficit), nearly all of that deficit will be filled by calories from bodyfat as it's being burned for energy. In this case, you'll still have plenty of energy for your workouts and your life in general because, besides the energy you'll get from your food intake, you'll be deriving energy from your bodyfat as it's being burned off. Your metabolism shouldn't be affected, because your body won't be too alarmed by a 500-calorie deficit. Of course, if you're a really small or a really lean person, your ideal calorie deficit for fat loss will be a little lower. On the other hand, if you're a larger person your deficit can be higher. But shooting for a 500-calorie deficit per day is a great strategy for fat-loss for most people. Those at the extreme ends in weight and bodyfat will want to go a little higher or a little lower than 500 calories for their deficit.

If you try for a larger deficit in order to hasten fat loss, the first thing you have to realize is that your body will slow your metabolism to try to save calories, which means in the future you'll have to reduce your calories even further to keep hitting the same deficit. For example, if you burn 2000 calories and eat only 1500 to create a 500-calorie deficit, you should be able to continue that pattern for quite some time and expect the same results – a one-pound fat loss per week. Your metabolism shouldn't slow much, if at all, when you stick to a 500-calorie deficit. However, if you burn 2000 calories and eat 1000 to create a 1000-calorie deficit, after a few weeks you'll probably need to eat just 700 to continue to create a 1000-calorie deficit. Why? Because eating so little will probably slow your metabolism to the point that you only burn 1700 per day, rather than the 2000 you burned per day before you caused your metabolism to slow down.

In this instance, one reason your metabolism will slow down is because your body will start burning it's own muscle tissue for an additional source of energy when your calorie deficit is too large. That means you won't burn as much bodyfat as you'd think you would looking at the size of your calorie deficit, because some of that energy deficit will be filled by the burning of lean tissue. Another reason your metabolism slows is that your body will begin to shut down the functioning of its nonessential systems when there are not enough calories available. Still *another* reason is the fact that your energy level will drop like a rock when you're not eating enough, which means you'll feel tired and lethargic and will burn fewer calories during activity.

So, getting back to the fat-burning "ceiling" question, the true "ceiling" to how much fat you can lose per day *is* greater than 500 calories' worth, but beyond that point you won't see 100% efficiency in bodyfat covering the calorie deficit. In other words, when you cut calories more than that you start losing part lean tissue and part bodyfat, but even more importantly, your metabolism will begin to slow, making fat loss that much harder in the future.

The solution to this dilemma is to face the physiological reality of the way the body responds, and that means you need to keep your calorie deficit within a certain limit on a daily basis. <u>You've got to relinquish the fantasy that you can lose a pound of fat or more per day.</u> It's just not going to happen – that's the honest truth.

Your next question might be, "Do I need to count calories to make sure I hit the right calorie deficit?" You'll be relieved to know that you don't need to literally count every calorie to make this concept of shooting for the appropriate calorie deficit work for you. If you are eating 3-6 relatively small but healthy meals (including a few treats here and there) and losing 0.5-3.0 pounds a week according to the scale (which will reflect a combination of fat loss and water loss from your diet), you will know that you're on track with the amount of food you're eating. Keep in mind, if you're a beginner you might not lose anything on the scale at first, even if you're losing bodyfat. It's common for beginners to build muscle and increase their capacity to store muscle glycogen during their first months of training. Beginners typically gain this lean weight during the first few months while losing bodyfat at the same time, which is why they might not show a gain or a loss in weight on the scale for the first month or two (in spite of the fact that they almost always lose bodyfat). Having your bodyfat percentage tested once a month and paying attention to how your clothes fit and how you look in the mirror should clue you in as to whether you're losing fat and on track.

As long as you're at least ten pounds above your ideal weight, another way to estimate your calorie deficit is to monitor hunger. If you're hitting the appropriate calorie deficit, you shouldn't be hungry between meals or snacks (assuming the majority of your diet consists of healthful foods), although you might start getting hungry an hour or so before it's time to eat again. If you're hitting the appropriate calorie deficit, you also should expect to wake up a bit hungry in the morning and find yourself looking forward to breakfast. In general, if you're hungry *all* the time your calorie deficit is probably too severe. However, if you're already lean (and got that way by dieting, not because you're naturally lean) and are looking to get even leaner, you should expect to be hungry pretty much all the time – it just goes with the territory of trying to get below your body's "set point," which is the weight and/or bodyfat percentage at which your body was designed to settle.

In spite of understanding this, you might be wondering about your friend who is thin as a rail and eats as much as he wants. You need to realize that there will always be those lucky few who are naturally very lean, and they usually won't feel hungry at all, even when they are nearly as lean as can be (these are the people who *wouldn't* survive if a true famine were to strike, because genetically they aren't programmed to carry much bodyfat and it's hard for them to sustain a calorie surplus – when they overeat their metabolic rate tends to rise automatically, which burns off the extra calories). And yes, you have permission to hate them for it!

Now that we've covered the "calorie deficit" aspect of fat loss, I'll explain another diet issue you'll need to address. The ideal energy balance as it relates to fat loss isn't only about the numbers at the end of the day (calories-in versus calories-out.) <u>Energy balance throughout different points in the day is just as important as energy balance at the end of the day if you are looking to lose fat rather than muscle and keep your metabolism up.</u> Even if you don't care about how much muscle you have per se, if you lose too much muscle you will pay the price of a lowered metabolism and will find yourself gaining weight even on tiny amounts of food. Besides, you'll never achieve a youthful, toned look if you don't have sufficient muscle mass.

The best thing to do in order to keep your energy balance in check throughout the day is to eat every three or four hours. Also, you should limit your workouts, particularly if they're intense ones, to one hour.

You might find it helpful to think of your calorie energy balance as a bank account. In this context, you can think of eating as "depositing" energy into your account. Daily living and exercise both "withdraw" energy, although daily living "withdraws" a small but steady amount, whereas exercise "withdraws" a big chunk at once. If you try to "withdraw" too much energy at once with a super-long exercise session, particularly if you haven't eaten recently, you might "bounce an energy check." Your body doesn't just quit on you by declaring "zero energy," since technically you'd be dead if nothing functioned at all. Instead, your survival mechanism kicks in as your energy reserves start running low. This causes a shift in hormones, which will downgrade your metabolism as you approach the point where you've run out of available energy. This downgrade in metabolism is a precaution your body takes so that you don't run your energy account completely dry. By conserving energy to a greater and greater extent the closer you get to running out, you will maintain just enough energy for quite a while so that, if it were a true famine, you'd be able to continue the search for food (again, which explains why many people can't keep their mind off food when they're dieting).

This downgrade in metabolism means you won't see the same weight loss benefit from a workout if you haven't been eating properly, because your body won't allow for the usual amount of energy to be burned during the workout. Also, if you haven't been eating properly your body will take steps to protect the most precious source of energy it has – your bodyfat. Of course, you can't perform *any* activity using no fuel at all, which means you'll surely begin to burn muscle if you burn too many calories at once or if you exercise when you haven't eaten enough in the past 24 hours. And, as you know, losing muscle always makes fat loss harder in the end.

If you could burn bodyfat quickly and in an unlimited amount, you could tap your excess bodyfat for fuel when you "bounce an energy check." However, that simply isn't possible from a physiological standpoint. There is a limit to the amount of bodyfat that your body can burn for energy in a given day. The reason for this limit goes back to the fact that your body reacts by trying to conserve energy when there aren't many calories coming in. By shifting the metabolism from primarily burning fat for fuel to primarily burning muscle, your body is acting smart in an energy crisis. Muscle burns extra calories every day, whereas fat does not. So, of course your body would rather burn muscle when it perceives an energy crisis, because less muscle means a lower metabolism, which means your body won't need as many calories in the future to maintain itself. When your calorie intake is low, burning muscle is the obvious choice to your body – the last thing your body wants to do is relinquish those precious fat stores that don't cost any energy to maintain and that it thinks is the only thing keeping you from starving to death.

How is all this information put to practical use? For one thing, it's not a good idea to exercise if you haven't eaten in the past three or four hours. However, if it makes you uncomfortable to eat before workouts, you should be okay exercising on an empty stomach as long as you eat well right after your workout and you keep your session to an hour or less. The reason you don't *have* to eat before your workout is that you should have glycogen stored in your muscles from previous meals. Glycogen stores won't take you as far as you could go if you also had a meal before exercising, but they should fuel you through 60-90 minutes of heavy training, assuming that you haven't been following a very-low-carb diet. However, if you haven't been eating many carbs you won't have much glycogen in storage, and you will be at risk for losing muscle if you exercise vigorously. On the other hand, easy cardio shouldn't be a problem in this situation because that type of exercise doesn't burn many calories, and the ones it does burn can come from bodyfat.

If you don't have any food calories or glycogen available for use and you complete a resistance-training session or an intense cardio workout, your body will be forced to burn your own muscle tissue for fuel. This is because bodyfat cannot be broken down into the glucose that is required to fuel those types of exercise, so in those instances your body has no choice but to break down muscle. During cardio, your body uses glucose (which can come from a recent meal, stored glycogen, or muscle tissue), fats circulating in your bloodstream from your last meal, and stored bodyfat for fuel. Resistance training is different, as it relies solely on carbs – that is, glucose and glycogen – for fuel.

You want to avoid the situation where you body is forced to break down muscle tissue for glucose. If you plan to exercise for over an hour at a time, you should have a solid meal during the 3-4 hours before your session, or else sip a sports drink or protein shake before or during your workout, especially if you're doing resistance training. You can get away with doing easy to moderate cardio with no food in your stomach, but you might find that you perform better if you've had something to eat.

I know that it sounds enticing to try and force your body to rely on bodyfat by not having any food calories in your system before exercise, but you have to understand that you'll lose weight either way, as long as you're running a calorie deficit on a daily basis. If you're running a calorie deficit, you will lose bodyfat even if you don't burn bodyfat specifically for your fuel during exercise. If this is a bit confusing, hang on – let me explain.

If you're using the food calories you've just eaten to fuel your exercise and you're also running a calorie deficit, there won't be any calories left over at the end of the day to be stored as bodyfat. Over the course of the day, all you need to do is expend more calories than you take in and you'll lose weight. It's not *what* you burn for energy (meaning food calories or calories from bodyfat), but rather *how much* energy you burn, that determines weight loss. Even if, theoretically, you could use bodyfat alone to fuel your exercise, that won't matter one bit if you proceed to consume more calories than you burn that day. Those extra food calories you'd be taking in will simply replace any of bodyfat you lost during exercise with "new" bodyfat if you overeat habitually. On the other hand, when you run a calorie deficit you will burn at least some bodyfat to cover that energy deficit, even if you don't do any exercise that day. You're probably getting sick of hearing this, but it all goes back to what I've been saying all along: You need to burn more calories than you consume in order to lose weight. Of course, the reason I say that you should avoid burning your own muscle for fuel is *not* because you won't lose weight (you'd still lose weight if you burn muscle, at least in the short-term), but because burning muscle will slow your metabolism, making weight loss in the future nearly impossible. And I refuse to give you a short-term fix that will allow you to lose weight initially, only to gain it all back before you know it.

Another application of seeking optimal energy balance throughout the day lies with the timing of exercise and the amount per session. If you split an hour-long workout into two 30-minute sessions, your energy balance will remain more consistent. By the same token, it's generally better to train for 30 minutes, six days per week rather than 60 minutes, three days per week. Applying this degree of scrutiny to your exercise schedule is getting very nit-picky for sure, but the reality is that training more frequently but with shorter sessions *is* optimal both from an energy balance standpoint and a hormonal standpoint. It also tends to be better from an intensity standpoint, because it's easier to work hard for just 30 minutes at a time.

How much does all of this specific stuff matter? Not very, especially when comparing people who exercise to people who don't. You get an enormous benefit simply by being one of the few who exercise the correct way, no matter how you split up the time, and when you get really picky with all the little details the improvements in results are miniscule, but you *will* realize them if you're willing to put in the extra effort and attention to detail. It's just that you start to see diminishing returns when you go beyond the point of simply training your entire body with weights plus some cardio three times a week, all other details aside. Most people aren't able or simply don't want to cater their lives to ideal exercise patterns all the time, and they still see great results.

The other reason it's okay to do longer but less frequent

sessions is that your muscles (if your diet is in order, and particularly if it's not too low in carbs) should have energy stored up in the form of muscle glycogen, meaning that you can "save" energy for the time when the "big check" (your workout) is "withdrawn." If you're a beginner or an intermediate-level exerciser, please don't concern yourself with splitting up your sessions. You don't need to bother with that level of detail yet. Save it for when you really need it if you hit a plateau down the line. Just get your sessions in and you will see the results. I include this information for the advanced exercisers reading, and also because I want to provide you with an overview on how all this fitness stuff works. I also don't want to withhold any of my "secrets" from you if you're willing to do everything possible to maximize your fitness success. Part of the key to long-term success, though, lies in not trying to do too much too soon. In other words, you want to KISS (keep it simple stupid) until *that* stops working, at which point you can try one of the more advanced or sophisticated methods. You always want to leave room to make changes in the future if you happen to plateau with what you're doing now. That way you should be able to continue making progress for a long time, without having to go through too much trouble before it's really necessary.

Although you can usually get away with "withdrawing" large amounts of energy all at once during a workout, it doesn't work that way when it comes to "depositing" energy by eating food. In other words, you can't consume all your calories for the day in the form of one huge meal and expect to see the same results you'd get if you ate five mini-meals spaced evenly throughout the day. This holds true for everyone, beginners included. You'll always get much better results from your exercise, especially in terms of changes in your appearance, if you eat properly. The reason that you can't eat all your calories at once and expect to stay lean has to do with the way the body responds to overfeeding and underfeeding. *Your body is designed to store energy, or calories, as bodyfat more efficiently than it burns bodyfat.* Your body would much rather store fat than burn it because bodyfat is a safety net for your survival during times when there isn't enough food around. Even though starving to death is probably one of the last things on your mind, all your body has to go by is your recent history of food intake. If you have been eating very little or skipping meals, your body must assume for the sake of its own survival that this state of affairs will probably continue. Your body will decide that it had better adapt and become more efficient at hoarding calories when you *do* provide them, or else you might die of starvation.

Let's take a look at the case where you eat one giant meal but have nothing else to eat that day. If you take in your full days' worth of calories all at once, you will be consuming more than your body can store as glycogen or burn as fuel right away. *Some* of the extra calories (specifically the calories from carbs) will go into glycogen stores in the muscles, which serve as a short-term storage place for fuel. In fact, if you have been weight training you will be able to store more of the carb calories as glycogen than someone who doesn't perform any resistance training. Only calories from carbohydrates can be stored as glycogen. The calories from fat and protein will be metabolized to perform various functions in the body. Once that need is met, any additional fat and protein calories will be burned for energy or converted to and stored as bodyfat – you can't store protein and fat in their original form for use in the immediate future like you can carbs.

Resistance training improves your body's ability to store carbs, as does choosing complex carbs over their refined counterparts. The ability to store more carbs is a good thing because that means fewer calories will be available to be converted into bodyfat. However, if your glycogen stores are topped off (depending on how in-shape he is, a 150-pound person can store 2000-3500 carb calories in the muscles) carbs too will be converted to and stored as bodyfat. In a nutshell, if you eat too many calories above maintenance, any of the three macronutrients can be stored as bodyfat. It's just that the carbs go towards replenishing muscle glycogen first before any of them will be converted into bodyfat. You still could eat enough calories from carbs to result in some being stored as bodyfat, but this would require eating thousands of calories above your maintenance level for days on end, which is a very hard thing to do. Most of the time when you're running a calorie surplus it's the dietary fat in your food that gets stored, while the carbs in the food go toward replenishing muscle glycogen. All this means that the only situation where you can overeat calories and not see an immediate increase in bodyfat is when you eat lots of low-fat, high-carb foods just for a day or two. This is the basis behind "carb-loading" athletes sometimes do, and also the low-fat diet craze of the 90s. Carb-loading has it's place if you follow a cyclic diet, but that issue is more appropriate for an advanced book on diet and nutrition. No matter how you slice it, though, if you eat too many calories on a regular basis you *will* gain bodyfat, and the most deadly combination is high-fat and high-carbs in the same meal (the foods we typically think of as "fattening" like casseroles and rich desserts).

One of the great things about exercise is that it burns glycogen, which prevents your glycogen stores from getting "topped off" (When your glycogen stores are topped off, you will gain bodyfat easily). Exercise also increases the capacity of your glycogen stores. Therefore, by burning glycogen and increasing glycogen storage capacity, exercise gives you a "safety net" that allows you to get away with overeating for a day or two without putting on bodyfat. On the other hand, sedentary individuals have a smaller capacity for glycogen storage that tends to be chronically topped off because they're not burning many calories during activity. This means almost any time they overeat, even if it's only by a little, they are apt to gain bodyfat.

If you make it easy by overeating habitually, your body tries to store as many calories as possible as bodyfat, because bodyfat is energy stored in reserve in case you hit another "famine" and go for too long without food. It's a pretty efficient energy reserve at that – each pound of bodyfat can provide about 3500 calories' worth of energy when it's burned. If you are a person who typically eats just two high-calorie meals per day, you might have an overall energy balance that looks okay (meaning that most days you land somewhere between maintenance and a 500-calorie deficit), but still have a high level of bodyfat. Although this might seem impossible at first glance, it happens because the more food you eat at once, the more likely it is to be stored as bodyfat and the less likely it is to be burned off or used to build or maintain muscle tissue and the other "nonessential" systems, including the immune system and the reproductive system. That's why people who don't eat properly tend to get sick more often and are more likely to experience reproductive problems. Even though a person who eats two large meals a day may be overweight, underweight, or at an ideal weight, if he's not spreading his food intake throughout the day his body will start to show signs of malnutrition. The body can't properly handle an overload of calories coming in at once. At the same time, it will suffer from not having enough food at other points during the day. Eating large meals that are spread too far apart is indeed a type of malnutrition because the proper nutrition isn't being provided at all times during the day.

Looking at this situation in the context of the bank accounts, if you skip breakfast, eat a light lunch, and then have a huge dinner, you end up trying to "withdraw" energy from an empty account all day ("bouncing checks" left and right), and you finally put all the "money" into the account at night when it's too late. Even though you can "save" some of that extra energy you're consuming as muscle glycogen to be used in the near future, some of it inevitably gets stored as bodyfat. Also, during the day when you're not eating enough to cover your energy "costs," your body slows down its rate of energy expenditure to accommodate the lack of available fuel. This results in a lower daily calorie burn. Your body might break down muscle tissue during this energy shortage, for a couple of reasons. Burning muscle provides a calorie source, for one thing. Also, muscle is "expensive" for your body to maintain calorie-wise. Your body knows that, in order to maintain the muscle, a good number of calories will be required on a daily basis. Your body isn't very confident that you will provide those calories if you've been going for long periods of time (due to blood sugar patterns after eating, "long periods of time" is about five hours) without food. If you go for too long between meals on a regular basis, your body won't be able to maintain much muscle, and less muscle means a lower daily calorie burn.

For all these reason and more, you aren't likely to lose bodyfat and you might even gain some if you eat just one or two big meals per day. You can't try to "save up" calories on a regular basis so that you can have a big meal and/or partake in drinking or eating sweets or fried food and expect to get or stay lean.

The bottom line is that you can enjoy a larger quantity of food *and* a reduced bodyweight if you eat small meals and snacks frequently throughout the day. Besides the fact that eating more food is satisfying and makes sticking to your diet plan easier, eating more is a good thing because a varied, nutritious diet will leave you healthier, happier, and more energetic, with more muscle and less fat on your body.

You should strive to keep your energy balance steady all day, meaning to keep a steady input versus output of calories. If you're trying to gain weight, just tweak your diet to have a slightly higher input of calories (about 250 extra calories per day, to the tune of 0.5 pound gained per week). If you're trying to lose weight, shift your diet to have a slightly higher output of calories (a deficit of 500 calories per day). If you want to maintain your weight, try to keep your calorie input and output the same.

An advanced exerciser who wants to gain muscle and lose fat while staying approximately the same weight over time might use some form of cyclic dieting. Assuming the person's goal is weight maintenance while gaining muscle and losing fat (commonly referred to as "toning"), during a cyclic diet energy intake versus output *won't* be equal on daily basis, but it *will* be equal over the period of a week, month, or year, depending on the length of the cycle. For instance, this type of plan might have you diet at a calorie deficit for four weeks followed by four weeks with a calorie surplus.

You can also use a cyclic diet plan for weight loss. A cyclic plan works great for those who want to maintain their muscle mass as they lose weight and bodyfat. An example of this type of plan is six weeks at a calorie deficit, followed by two weeks at maintenance or a calorie surplus in order to re-set metabolism and rebuild any muscle that was lost while dieting. Although cyclic diets are always an option, for a beginner or for someone getting back into an exercise routine, muscle gain and/or fat loss should be fairly easy to accomplish without having to do anything other than be in a calorie surplus or run a calorie deficit on a daily basis.

Even if you're an intermediate or advanced exerciser, if you just want to maintain your shape or see gradual improvement over time, all you really need to do is eat when you're hungry and stop when you're full. Just be sure to choose nutritious foods the majority of the time (See Reference B in the back of the book for nutrition guidelines for exercisers).

No matter what your particular goals, everyone needs a steady supply of calories and protein to keep his metabolism humming and to rebuild muscle tissue after it gets broken down during weight training. If your diet doesn't contain enough of the nutrient "building blocks" your muscles need, you simply won't see the same results from your resistance training, no matter how hard you work out. After all, you can't build muscle from nothing ("nothing" meaning not enough protein and total calories in the diet to meet energy demands with enough left over for muscle building). And, if you fail to eat enough carbohydrates, your liver and muscle glycogen will remain chronically depleted. When you fail to replenish glycogen to at least moderate levels, you'll get mediocre results from your exercise program because you won't recover as fast or as thoroughly. Also, if you're running low on carbs you will tend to feel drained of energy and strength during your workouts. This means you won't burn as many calories during your exercise sessions and you won't lose as much bodyfat. You'll also be more likely to injure yourself if you work out while following a very-low-carb diet because your muscles won't be holding as much water and glycogen, both of which serve as structural supports for the tissues. All of these factors will hold you back in your workout intensity and your recovery rate, both of which will slow your overall progress. This is why very low-carb diets aren't the best solution for the person whose primary goal is to get in great shape. Strictly for weight-loss purposes, there's no doubt that low-carb diets work very well for some people, and particularly those with problems controlling blood sugar, but low-carb diets certainly aren't ideal for exercise performance.

If you want the weight loss, steady blood sugar, and appetite control that many experience while eating low-carb without suffering from a lack of workout intensity, you can get around the dilemma by using a week-long cyclic diet plan where you have more carbs on some days and less on others. Another option is to eat carbs before and/or after your workout, but avoid or limit them at other times. When you follow a plan that includes carbohydrates only at specific times, you get to enjoy the accelerated fat loss that goes along with a reduced calorie and carb intake, while at the same time maintaining the ability to satisfy cravings and have plenty of strength and stamina for your workouts. Your intense workouts should be scheduled around the days when your carb intake or glycogen levels are higher. You should do your less taxing workouts on the low-carb days, and especially your moderate-pace cardio since that type of exercise can tap into bodyfat stores for fuel.

There are many factors that go into the design of a carb-cycling plan, and if you choose to follow one it's very important that your workout and diet schedule coincide in a specific manner for best results. These plans need to be designed on an individual basis because there are so many factors to consider, and I'm not going to discuss anything beyond generalized diet advice in this book. I hope to write a separate book on nutrition for exercisers in the future. Until then, please visit my website, www.homeexercisecoach.com or give me a call if you'd like to set up an appointment to delve in specific diet recommendations and create a plan (perhaps a carb-cycling one) personalized to your needs. Carb-cycling is an advanced technique that is usually most appropriate after you've already lost the majority of your excess bodyfat through a classic calorie-controlled diet and exercise plan that includes weights and cardio. Carb-cycling diets are usually not necessary until you've reached the point where you only have about 10 pounds of bodyfat left to lose, not because they don't work in other cases, but because they're usually not worth the hassle, planning, and regimentation involved until the traditional methods stop working for you. However, some people don't do well using traditional methods and might want to try a carb-cycling plan right off the bat, so keep it in mind if you're having trouble losing weight and/or bodyfat with the method you're using now.

When I talk about carbohydrates in the diet, realize that it's not just grains and sugar I'm referring to. Fruits, veggies, dairy, and nuts all contain some carbs, and if you don't have a particularly active job and/or you're not exercising nearly every day, these foods alone will probably provide you with plenty of carbs to fuel your workouts. In this case, a diet containing multiple servings of fruits and vegetables per day would already be considered a "moderate-carb" plan, even if it didn't include any grains or sugar. On the other hand, if your job is labor-intensive and/or you exercise for at least an hour nearly every day, a diet with fruits and vegetables as the only source of carbs would be considered a very-low-carb diet. Carbohydrate requirements are contingent upon activity levels. In general, nutritional needs for relatively active people are different from nutritional needs of sedentary or moderately active people. In Reference B you'll find a summary of important nutrition issues for exercisers.

For a moment, I'd like to return to the point that it's better to eat small portions and eat frequently. Above and beyond the positive effect this has on exercise results and performance, providing your body with a steady supply of food will go a long way toward reducing your bodyfat percentage. In many cases, making the change to eating the right foods in the right quantities every few hours will make more of a difference than exercise when it comes to stripping off bodyfat! Of course, exercise does wonders and is an important piece of the puzzle for reducing bodyfat. The good news is that a steady supply of food happens to work synergistically when combined with exercise – it's really the two together that have such an incredibly powerful effect on the way you look and feel.

As you may have begun to deduce by this point, if you want to lose weight it really doesn't matter whether you burn more calories from activity to create your calorie deficit or whether you cut out the calories from your diet instead. Now, this doesn't mean that you don't need to exercise at all, because <u>exercise has positive effects on your metabolism above and beyond the number of calories burned while exercising</u>. Exercise also improves nutrient partitioning, which means that your body starts to put more incoming calories toward muscle building and maintenance, leaving fewer calories available to be stored as bodyfat. Completing at least 2-3 weight-training and cardio sessions per week will allow you to reap the benefits of exercise on your body composition (the amount of lean weight compared to the amount of bodyfat you carry). You need to spend about 30 minutes on weight training and 30 minutes on cardio 2-3 days per week to enjoy the full benefits of improved nutrient partitioning and body composition. At the same time, these 2-3 workouts per week also have influence on the calorie-burning end. Exercise encourages your body to burn calories from bodyfat instead of muscle when it has to tap into stored energy for fuel.

Additional exercise beyond this minimum recommendation will burn extra calories and allow you to build even more muscle, but will only be useful for weight management if you're having trouble manipulating your diet to create that 500-calorie energy deficit. Most people would rather run 30 minutes and have just 1 cup of pasta at dinner than run 60 minutes and have 2 cups (the 250 calories you can save by having 1 cup of pasta instead of 2 is about the same that you'd burn running an extra 30 minutes). If you would rather do the extra exercise in order to be able to eat more, that's fine, but just keep in mind that you might be putting yourself at risk for injuries, exhaustion, burnout, and overtraining syndrome (you can read more about overtraining syndrome in Strategy 29).

Of course, some people have physique goals that reach beyond basic weight maintenance and health. Only if you truly aspire to reach the very top level of fitness, complete with a ripped, head-turning body (and you're willing and able to work hard and sacrifice for it) is it necessary to do all of that extra training *on top* of having a great diet. If you want bulging muscles or a ripped six-pack, you may have to do much more than 2-3 hours a week – unless you have incredible genetics, you'll have to do 1-2 hours a day. For the average person that just wants to look good and be fit while still having a life outside the gym, maintaining a good diet allows you to "get away" with spending less time exercising and still get the results you want.

Before you think you'll never have time to reach a high level of fitness, realize that there are other ways to increase your calorie burn and improve nutrient partitioning besides spending more time exercising. You must be aware that certain *types* of exercise result in a greater number of calories burned over the 24-hour period following your workout session.

What most people don't know about moderate cardiovascular activity such as walking is that this type of exercise (steady-pace cardio) only burns calories *during the time you are actually performing the activity*, whereas there are other types of exercise that have a metabolism-boosting effect *for the entire 24-hour period following your workout*. While the number of calories burned during your exercise session is important, it's more effective for weight management and bodyfat loss to do exercise that also generates a post-exercise calorie burn. See, the calories burned *during* a typical exercise session aren't going to be significant enough to result in very much weight loss, especially when compared to the number of calories contained in food. For instance, a 180-pound person burns about 200 calories walking for a 30 minutes at 4 m.p.h. (this is a pretty good clip – most people break into a jog at 5 m.p.h.). Unfortunately, eating a couple of small cookies or ¾ of a candy bar will put those 200 calories right back into your body, leaving you back where you started calorie-wise. So you will get much more "bang" for your exercise "buck" if you perform more of the types of exercise that boost your metabolism for an entire day. This will allow you to burn much more fat than if you just stick to steady-pace cardio.

If you raise your metabolism by using specific techniques such as performing the metabolism-boosting types of exercise, you might not even have to do *any* steady-pace cardio in order to lose weight and keep it off. That means you can enjoy fat loss without having to endure hour-long aerobics classes, 5-mile jogs, or long, sweaty sessions on the stairmaster. And if you *do* opt to partake in steady-pace cardio, you will know that all the work is going toward a loss of bodyfat, because you will have already created an energy deficit even before the additional cardio is taken into consideration.

Now, we'll take a look at which exercises fall into this category, as well as the seven most important things you can do to raise your metabolism, either by increasing your daily calorie needs or by preventing a drop in your metabolic rate.

The 7 Keys to Raising Your Metabolism for Life

As a fitness professional with countless hours of research and experience under my belt helping clients re-shape their bodies, I have formulated a recipe for success in the quest for achieving a fit, tight body. It consists of seven components you should strive to incorporate into your life if you want to get and stay lean. After you have studied these principles, you will be ready for the Strategy sections of this book where you will pick up tips to help you apply them. The Strategy sections will serve as a guide to help you form your goals, and are designed to ensure that you're able to apply what you're learning to your life.

I think you'll agree that it's not enough just to know *what* to do – many people know what they *should* do, but if they don't *actually follow through and do it*, what's the point? Likewise, all the discipline and ambition in the world won't do you any good if you don't know what's effective and what's not. Most of the books on health, fitness, and dieting that I've seen focus either on information (what you *should* do) or on motivation/behavior modification (how to get yourself to actually *do it*). This System is different because it brings these two critical pieces together, and both are imperative to your success.

This section covers the "7 Keys," which spell out exactly what you need to do to raise your metabolism. It also explains (in everyday language) why these methods work. The information contained in this section will cut through all the confusing advice to clearly reveal which actions and goals will lead to the results you're after. All the goals that lead to success in health, fitness and weight loss will align with these seven principles of metabolism in some manner. If you follow them, you are sure to develop a lean, fit and healthy body.

Key 1: <u>Progressive</u> resistance training

Resistance training is an umbrella term for exercises using free weights or weight-stack machines and exercises using your bodyweight as resistance (such as push-ups). You *must* perform compound exercises (those that involve movement across multiple joints and utilize more than one muscle group) for both the upper and lower body if you're serious about stimulating your metabolism. Compound exercises are most effective when performed to near or absolute muscular failure, meaning that the weight is heavy enough to cause your muscles to give up at or before you've completed 15 repetitions (reps) with correct form. The metabolism-boosting compound exercises include squats, deadlifts, leg press, and lunges for the lower body, and chest press, shoulder press, pulldowns, and rows for the upper body.

Isolation exercises are those that involve movement across only one joint and target just one muscle at a time. These exercises (such as a bicep curl) can be useful for maximizing the development of individual muscles. However, isolation exercises aren't the most efficient or effective way to develop a base of lean body mass, which is the most important factor for your metabolism. Isolation exercises also won't do much for your appearance if you have a layer of fat covering your muscles. It's the compound exercises that will lead to a leaner body the quickest. When you do compound exercises you can lift relatively heavier weights because more than one muscle group is involved – meaning you get faster results. And, since compound exercises are so intense and use so many muscles at once, a full-body routine doesn't take very long to do, yet it burns lots of calories and helps reduce bodyfat. That will leave you with more time to spend on cardio if you choose, which will accelerate your loss of bodyfat.

Compound exercises offer another bonus for dieters – performing them helps you maintain muscle and bone tissue while you're dieting. Each pound of muscle you build will burn about 35 extra calories per day (1). That's the reason why men can usually eat more than women without putting on bodyfat – they carry more muscle, and consequently require more calories. Athletes, who tend to be more muscular than the average person, also eat a high number of calories and stay lean. If you lose muscle while dieting, your daily calorie needs (your maintenance calorie level) goes down, making it harder to lose weight. Think how much easier it would be to create your 500-calorie deficit if you could build more muscle! If you build and maintain just five pounds of muscle, every day whether you exercise or not you will burn at least 175 extra calories. That's the same calorie burn you'd get from taking nearly a two-mile walk, *every day*. That sure makes dieting easier!

For your resistance training, be sure to focus on the compound movements, since they use the most muscle tissue. You should choose a weight that allows you to perform 8-12 repetitions with correct form before your muscle gives up. In some cases you might go with more or less reps – anything from 3 reps up to 20 reps has its place at times. You can't go wrong with 8-12, though, because that range has been proven over and over to produce results. Just keep in mind that, in general, it's better to choose a heavier weight than it is to keep increasing reps, especially once you're able to complete 15 reps with good form using a particular weight. If you have been lifting consistently for at least three months, you should make sure to lift in the 5-8-rep range at times. Mixing up your workouts ensures that you won't get stuck in a training rut where you make little or no progress.

Once you're at the point where you're completely happy with the way you look and feel, you can simply continue performing the same workouts you've been doing to maintain your fitness level. However, if you want to continue to reduce bodyfat and raise your metabolism further, you'll need to keep pushing yourself. Even if you haven't been able to manage 15 reps with a certain weight, try a heavier weight anyway after a month or two. You might surprise yourself – when you go back to the original weight you'll probably get more reps than you did before. That's because your muscles will be forced to adapt to the new weight, which makes the lighter weights feel so much easier.

It's especially important to work the legs, butt, and back during resistance training because they are the largest muscles in the body and consequently will increase your metabolism the most when you exercise them. Don't make the mistake of skipping lower body exercises when you do your resistance training just because you "work" your legs with cycling or running. Cardio doesn't train the muscles the same way as resistance training – no matter how much cardio you do or how vigorously you do it, you still need to perform the compound lifts for your legs. If you're training really hard with cardio you will probably need to limit your resistance training to two full-body workouts per week to avoid overtraining, but you definitely want to hit all of your muscles with resistance training at least twice per week.

As you develop and condition your muscles by doing resistance training, the fat will start melting away and you will be left with a tight, toned, and shapely physique. As an added bonus, by developing the key areas through the proper weight-training program your body will begin to burn more calories every day. This saves you from having to go on a super-strict diet or from having to endure hours of cardio to keep the fat off. And just when you thought it couldn't get any better, wait until you hear this: Resistance training improves your body's ability to handle carbohydrates. When you have been faithful to a resistance-training routine your body gets better at taking glucose into the muscles to be stored as glycogen, which means there's less of a chance there will be any calories left over to be converted into bodyfat. You'll also find that your blood sugar level is steadier when you've been doing resistance training, which leads to higher and more consistent energy levels, fewer food cravings, a lower risk for developing diabetes, and less abdominal fat.

Also, don't forget that you'll want to have a firm body once the bodyfat you're targeting starts to come off. The most common result people want out of exercise is weight loss, but that's followed closely behind by "toning." "Toning" simply means an increase in muscle size and a decrease in bodyfat. Besides simply building muscle and helping you reduce bodyfat, however, resistance training makes you smaller at a given weight, since muscle is quite a bit denser than fat. In fact, 10 pounds of fat takes up the same amount of space as 17 pounds of muscle (2). As long as you keep up with your resistance training, you will fit into smaller clothing sizes even if you don't lose weight. Of course, if you *do* lose weight while staying consistent with your resistance-training routine you'll be much, much smaller! You'll look more compact, tight, and sleek all the time if you keep up with your resistance training. Both men and women look better when they weight-train in conjunction with dieting – most people don't find skin and bones to be very attractive.

Even if you think you have plenty of muscle already, if you're successful with fat loss you will inevitably end up losing some muscle along the way. The only weapon you have to guard against that process is resistance training. And remember, besides the fact that muscle is what gives your body a toned look, muscle tissue burns lots of calories every day to maintain itself (whereas excess bodyfat burns virtually none). The most important key to your long-term weight-loss success is to maintain as much muscle as possible while dieting. And ladies, don't worry – it's extremely rare to find a women who has anything close to the hormonal makeup necessary to build a "manly" or "bulky" physique, especially when she's also doing cardio and following a weight-loss diet. Even if a woman *does* have the ability to build lots of muscle, unless she's eating above maintenance calories she won't gain an ounce. When a female performs resistance training, it simply helps her develop feminine curves and it raises her metabolism, helping her keep the fat off for good.

Resistance training is the best weapon you have for firming and re-shaping your body. The heavier and more intensely you weight-train, the faster you'll re-shape your body, and the greater your post-workout calorie burn will be. Intensity can be achieved in a number of different ways, the most straightforward being the amount of weight used during resistance training. The post-workout calorie burn I've been talking about can last for up to 24 hours after the workout, and if you work hard enough to trigger it, you'll burn more calories than you normally would all day and night, even while you're sleeping. Keep in mind, the post-workout calorie burn is *in addition to* the calories burned during the actual workout, and of course the calories burned during the actual workout will be higher the harder you work during your weight training.

Key 2: Stabilize blood sugar levels by eating meals and snacks containing protein, carbs, and fat every few hours

The importance of this key for getting lean cannot be overstated. Eating small meals and snacks every few hours works like a charm to improve health, productivity, mood, muscle tone, energy level, and bodyfat percentage. That's just a short list of the benefits, by the way.

Ideally you want each meal, mini-meal, or snack to contain a significant amount of each macronutrient (the three macronutrients are protein, carbs, and fat). It's not necessary to keep any specific macronutrient ratio – as long as you get some of each in most of your meals and snacks you should be fine. You might be familiar with the "Zone" diet, which requires that 40% of calories in each meal or snack come from carbs, 30% come from fat, and 30% come from protein. As it turns out, the "Zone" also dictates the number of calories to eat. The relatively low calorie level is really the reason the diet works, at least in the beginning. The problem with the Zone is that calories are set at such a low level that your metabolism is likely to slow, which is the reason why many people plateau pretty quickly on that plan.

Even though it's not important that each meal or snack contain a particular macronutrient ratio, it *is* important that you consume enough of the essential nutrients each day to keep your metabolism running at maximum efficiency. One of the essentials is protein. To maximize metabolism, dieters should consume at least 1 gram of protein per pound of bodyweight each day.

To see how this recommendation relates to food, I'll use a skinless chicken breast half (4 oz. of chicken) as an example. 4 oz. of chicken breast contains about 25 grams of protein. If you weigh 150 pounds and are dieting, you need 150 grams of protein (1 gram x 150 pounds) a day. Each gram of protein contains 4 calories, so the 25 grams of protein in the chicken contributes 100 calories from protein to the diet (25 grams x 4 calories per gram = 100). You need 600 calories from protein per day to meet the guideline (150 pound person x 1 gram of protein per pound x 4 calories per gram = 600).

Besides protein, the only real *macronutrient* requirement for your health is that you get your essential fatty acids (EFAs). Many people choose to supplement to be sure they get enough EFAs on a regular basis. Fish oil capsules fit the bill here – 3-6 grams per day should do the trick. I recommend leaning toward six when you're dieting because EFAs, although they are a fat themselves, facilitate the burning of bodyfat, especially when you're running a calorie deficit. EFAs also offer a host of other health benefits. Although protein and EFAs are the only macronutrients that you *must* include in your diet to stay healthy (since your body can't produce those compounds on it's own), you still need to maintain the correct energy balance and get all the necessary *micronutrients* (vitamins and minerals). That means you're going to need other sources of calories besides protein and EFAs. In case you were wondering, consuming *more* protein and EFAs beyond the recommended amount won't do much of anything. In other words, it's not ideal to get *all* your calories from protein and EFAs, and in fact it would be harmful to do so because you wouldn't be getting all the important micronutrients found in other food groups. Once you meet your protein and EFA requirements, you should obtain the rest of your calories from other sources.

To figure out how many calories you require each day to reach your goals, you need to start by finding your maintenance calorie level. You might know (or be able to estimate) this number if you've counted calories in the past. If you've never tracked your calories closely, you can estimate your maintenance calorie level using an easy formula. Simply find your daily activity level and the amount of exercise you do in the chart on the next page, then take your total body weight and multiply it by the number indicated in the chart.

Daily Activity level*	Exercise	Multiplier**
Sedentary	0-2 hours per week	10 x TBW
Sedentary	2-6 hours per week	12 x TBW
Sedentary	6+ hours per week	14 x TBW
Moderately active	0-2 hours per week	12 x TBW
Moderately active	2-6 hours per week	14 x TBW
Moderately active	6+ hours per week	16 x TBW
Very active	0-2 hour per week	14 x TBW
Very active	2-6 hours per week	16 x TBW
Very active	6+ hours per week	18 x TBW

*Daily activity level does not include exercise.
**Adjust up 1 or 2 points for males and for lean individuals.
Adjust down 1 or 2 points for females and those with a high bodyfat %.

    The number you get should approximate your maintenance calorie level per day. These numbers are estimates at best, so it's still a good idea to track your calorie intake for at least a week. If you track your calorie intake for a week, it will allow you to pinpoint the calorie level that you require to maintain your weight. Once you find your "real" maintenance calorie level by monitoring your diet, you can find your own personal multiplier by dividing your maintenance calorie level by your weight. Generally, if your multiplier varies from the table above it's usually because you don't have an "average" bodyfat percentage. That means the multiplier in the table might be one or two numbers too high for people who have a higher bodyfat percentage, and one or two numbers too low for people who have a lower bodyfat percentage. Because women tend to have a higher bodyfat percentage than men, adjust your multiplier according to your gender and your build if you choose to estimate your maintenance calorie level by using the numbers in the table.

    Once you know or have an estimate of your maintenance calorie level, you might need to add or subtract calories from that figure to find the number that you should shoot for per day. Whether you add calories or subtract them will depend on your goals. If your primary goal is fat loss, you should subtract 500 calories from your maintenance calorie level. That will allow for the 500-calorie deficit recommended for fat loss. Add 250 to your maintenance number if your primary goal is to build muscle. This will put you in the calorie surplus that is recommended for muscle gain. If you don't want to change your weight and aren't going to use a cyclic diet, you should stick with your maintenance calorie level.

Once you know how many calories to consume each day, take 20-30% of that number. That's the approximate number of calories you should obtain from dietary fat. Each gram of fat contains 9 calories, so by dividing the calories from fat by 9 you can figure out how many grams of fat to shoot for. For instance, if you need 2000 calories per day to reach your goals, 20-30% of 2000 calories is 400-600 calories. If you divide 400-600 by 9, you'll find that you should consume 44-66 grams of fat per day. Going back to the chicken breast example, 4 oz. of skinless chicken breast contains about 3 grams of fat, or 27 calories from fat (3 grams x 9 calories per gram = 27). Keep in mind, your EFAs need to be included as part of your fat intake, even if you take them in pill form (each 1000mg (1 gram) pill contains 1 gram of fat or 9 calories).

If you've been following along, you should have already figured out how many calories to obtain from protein (you want 1 gram per pound of bodyweight, and each gram of protein contains 4 calories). After you know how many calories to obtain from protein and how many to obtain from fat, add those two figures together and then subtract that number from your total calories per day. This shows you how many calories you have left after you've met the guidelines for protein and fat. After you've met your protein and fat requirements, the rest of your calories for the day can come from carbohydrates, including those found in whole grains, fruits, vegetables, nuts, legumes, dairy products, and any refined grains or sugars you consume. If you have alcohol or "non-impact carbs" like fiber, glycerol, or sugar alcohols, include those calories as part of your calories from carbs, simply because they clearly aren't proteins or fats, and those calories still need to be counted toward your daily total. Many protein bars and "low-carb" products will have these "non-impact carbs." The carbs in these products are called "non-impact" because they don't increase your blood sugar level like most carbs do, but they still provide calories to the body. That's why the calories don't always add up if you do the math on some of those protein bars. That is, if you take the carbohydrate grams listed on the label multiplied by 4, add that to the protein grams multiplied by 4, and add that to the fat grams multiplied by 9, the calorie total you get might be lower than the total calories listed on the product. By the time of this printing, the non-impact carbs don't have to be listed in the carb count from a legal standpoint, although this can be misleading because "non-impact" carbs still contribute calories to the food.

When choosing your meals and snacks, your best bet is to choose carbohydrates of the complex variety, which, along with eating every few hours, keeps your blood sugar regulated and your glucose metabolism in top-notch condition. The fiber in the complex carbs, along with including moderate amounts of protein and fat in each meal or snack, will help slow digestion. This keeps insulin under control, which helps reduce bodyfat. Including protein, fat, and fiber in each meal also keeps you feeling full longer so you won't be starving again an hour or two after you eat. Eating frequently also helps control hunger – if you eat every few hours, you should never get so ravenously hungry that you lose control. <u>Dieters actually should eat more frequently than those who just want to maintain their weight.</u> This is because dieters need to take extra precaution against the plummeting energy level and hunger pains that are more likely to occur when you're running a calorie deficit.

Although eating more frequently tends to promote diet compliance because it helps fight hunger, you might find that sticking to just three meals per day works well for you (notice that I didn't say one or two meals!) If you stick to "3 squares" and are happy with the results, there's no reason to force yourself to eat more often. However, if you've been doing three meals and still have stubborn areas on your body that haven't firmed up, or you find that you're otherwise hitting a plateau, consider eating more often for a trial period to see if it makes a difference. Also, if you find your energy level flagging or your fat loss slowing to a crawl, it might be time to try eating more often. This could mean 4-6 mini-meals per day, or three meals and a couple of snacks. All you really need to do to get your 4-6 "meals" is have a little less food at your three main meals and add two between-meal snacks, which can be a nutrition bar or nutrition shake. Many people find that the extra energy and faster rate of fat loss are worth the inconvenience of having to eat more often. With all the meal replacement products out there today (you can even buy them at convenience stores now), finding convenient sources of nutrition isn't very difficult at all. If you choose to rely on some of these nutrition products, sample a variety of brands and flavors to figure out which ones you like and then order them in bulk to save money. Experiment to find the number of meals and snacks that works best for you. Keep in mind that the leaner you get, the more tinkering you may need to do if you want to keep pushing for more fat loss.

Key 3: Perform 3-5 cardio workouts per week

Some people like it and most people hate it, but to lose weight faster you simply must do it! Cardio helps with fat loss in a myriad of ways. It burns calories, resulting in pounds lost as long as your diet is in order. Cardio helps regulate blood sugar and appetite. Dieters that perform cardio also tend to maintain more lean body mass (when the cardio is done in reasonable amounts, which I will define shortly). Cardio also promotes the mobilization and loss of bodyfat. These things are true of cardio in general, but high-intensity cardio is clearly superior for losing bodyfat, especially toward the end of a diet. <u>If you are looking at the last 10-20 pounds of a diet, all else being equal, you will always lose faster and be leaner if you perform interval training or some other type of high-intensity cardiovascular workout.</u>

Interval training consists of alternating periods of recovery-pace cardio (such as a 3-m.p.h. flat walk) with periods of all-out effort (such as a sprint). If you do this type of training, you can crank up your metabolism to get that post-exercise calorie burn, similar to what happens when you weight-train. In addition, you will burn more calories per minute of exercise with interval training than you ever could with steady-pace cardio.

Before you get too excited by all the calorie-blasting possibilities, know that high-intensity training is not something you should undertake every day. You can do one or two all-out cardio workouts per week for up to six weeks at a time before you should take a month off from such strenuous activity. If you choose to do more than two cardio workouts per week in total, the rest of your workouts should be easy to moderate-intensity.

Shoot for 3-5 cardio workouts per week (20-60 minutes each) if you want to make a significant difference in the number of calories you burn per day. 20 minutes is fine if you're doing cardio primarily for heart health, but spend longer if your purpose is to increase your rate of weight loss. The 3-5 days is a recommendation, but not a requirement – one or two days is so much better than none (you *don't* want to think, "If I can't do five days it isn't worth it to do any at all). If you are looking to increase your metabolism as much as you can, you should push yourself during the 1-2 intense workouts you're "allowed" per week. One of your intense workouts might be a 30-minute bike ride pedaling as vigorously as you can, and another could be the interval sprints described above. Supplement this work with up to three lower-intensity cardio sessions, which might include one moderate-pace bike ride, one brisk walk, and one easy to moderate-intensity session on the stairmaster at the gym, for example.

The better you can condition your cardiovascular system, the more calories you will be able to burn during your cardio, which will help with fat loss. Cardio also promotes fat loss for another reason – it increases circulation to the peripheral regions of the body. The increased circulation helps to mobilize fat in the "stubborn areas" so that it can be burned for energy. In females, the stubborn fat deposits are typically found on the hips and thighs, while in males they are typically found on the stomach and low back. These fat deposits are referred to as "stubborn" because even individuals who are at their ideal weight and bodyfat percentage can still have excess fat in these areas. Also, the body quite often will start burning muscle before it will burn off the "stubborn" fat deposits, unless you know how to circumvent this problem. Cardio, and especial high-intensity interval training, is the best weapon you have for tackling stubborn fat deposits. Reducing carbohydrate intake and alcohol intake is the second-best weapon you have for fighting stubborn fat deposits.

To understand more about burning fat, you have to know that there are two types of fat that are important to human metabolism. Visceral fat is the fat deep inside your body that is found surrounding your organs. Too much visceral fat can make your stomach look bloated or distended. Visceral fat is usually the first to go on a diet, even if you're not doing cardio. There is an exception to this rule, though, and it applies to steroid and andro users. The reason is that testosterone tends to increase the ratio of visceral fat to subcutaneous fat. Subcutaneous fat, the second type, is the fat lying just underneath the skin. Cardio tends to burn the subcutaneous fat that is harder to take off just by dieting. Not only does cardio help with weight loss by burning calories in general, but it also helps to facilitate the mobilization of bodyfat, particularly in stubborn areas that diet and weight training alone won't always address. See, even if you are running a calorie deficit, if you don't mobilize the fat molecules so they can leave the fat cells to be burned for energy you won't lose bodyfat – you'll burn muscle instead. Cardio helps to circumvent this problem.

As long as you aren't significantly overweight, the most effective cardiovascular activities for weight loss are the ones that burn the most calories per minute. Climbing (both hills and stairs), a vigorous effort on an elliptical cross-trainer, and running fall into this category. Bicycling and walking are better choices for the significantly overweight and for beginners. If you are just starting an exercise program, it's a good idea to stick to bicycling, flat or 1-5% incline-walking, or an elliptical trainer on an easy setting until you have developed a base of cardiovascular fitness. Once you've established a foundation, you can build up to higher intensities if desired. People who are just starting out get so much out of just doing *something* that you should take advantage and move, but don't push yourself to the limit. As a beginner, you don't need to do that in order to see results, and it's not even healthy to tax yourself to that degree at this point. Just get yourself into a routine and you *will* eventually achieve all your goals.

Key 4: Pursue active recreation

If you spend your free time engaging in active pursuits, you will burn extra calories and have fun at the same time. What could be easier? Watching TV and sitting at the computer are the worst things you can do for your waistline (actually, eating junk food at the same time would be worse, but you get the idea).

If you don't already partake, think of things you used to do as a kid or that you have done in the past and make these activities a regular habit. Bring a friend or family member along to enjoy the activity with you. Skiing, pickup basketball, hiking, tennis, gardening, and leisurely bike rides are just a few of your options. Do you have any other ideas? You will burn lots of calories and have tons of fun. Another thing you might consider is completing household jobs like mowing the lawn, walking the dog or shoveling the driveway yourself instead of handing off that chore to a family member or hiring someone to do it. You can earn some brownie points or save a few bucks and burn some serious calories at the same time.

Sports are another fun way to become more active. Find an adult intramurals program or join a team! You'll be so focused on the game and so pumped up on adrenaline that you will hardly notice when you start breaking a sweat! Before you know it, you'll have blasted hundreds of calories without thinking too much about it.

Key 5: On the job (or at home), move!

Whenever you have a choice, always choose movement. When there are boxes to be carried or errands that can be run on foot, be the first to volunteer. If you are talking on the phone, stand up and walk around the room instead of sitting. Park in the furthest spot away from the entrance to a store, not in the closest! Someone else will love to find that close spot, and you know that you could use the extra walking. It's funny that in today's world every effort is made to do less physical work – and look where it got us! Over half of American adults are overweight. Yikes! In our relentless pursuit of convenience and ease of living, we have made ourselves as a society sick and unhealthy.

Walking for leisure, playing with your kids, or walking the dog are other ways to boost your calorie burn for the day. These activities won't help your system upgrade its metabolism like the tougher cardio unless you are extremely out of shape, but they *will* burn extra calories, and every little bit helps when you're trying to lose weight. You're also less likely to snack when you keep moving, because you're kept busy for one thing, but also because physical activity leads to the release of endorphins, which make you feel good and therefore less likely to eat when you're not hungry.

Key 6: Consider supplements

Although many supplements make outrageous claims regarding the muscle gain or fat loss you will experience if you take them, supplements offer the most value when they are used to correct vitamin and mineral deficiencies. <u>Did you know that a deficiency in any vitamin or mineral sets you up for a metabolic slowdown</u>? All the processes the body depends on to function at its peak require that the essential vitamins and minerals be available in sufficient quantity, sometimes on a daily basis. For instance, the water-soluble vitamins cannot be stored in the body for any significant length of time. If you don't get the right amounts on a daily basis, your body *will* suffer the consequences. If you think this can't be affecting you, realize that some people have felt "sick" for so long that it feels normal to them! They don't realize why they can't seem to get going without their giant cup of coffee, why they want to lie on the couch watching TV all day, or why they can't seem to muster up the energy to exercise. Although there is no "magic" supplement that burns fat like crazy, never underestimate the power of optimizing your body's functioning. If you eat nutritious foods, supplement as needed, and exercise, your body will respond more favorably than if you neglected to do those things but took all the weight-loss drugs in the world.

Unfortunately, it's hard to get all the necessary micronutrients from your diet no matter how "healthy" you eat, although in the past they were readily available in our food. Most of our food today has been stripped of its vitamins and minerals by all the food processing. Sometimes food companies add synthetic vitamins and minerals to their foods to try to make up for what is missing. "Enriched" products are made in this way. The "enriched" products will never be as nutritious as fresh, unprocessed food, but unfortunately high-quality, nutritious food is harder and harder (and much more expensive when you look to organic products, which aren't necessarily more nutritious) to come by these days. A multivitamin/mineral can go a long way toward setting you straight. A generic brand right from the pharmacy or supermarket will be your most economical (and still effective) option, but it's true that you will tend to get a slightly better rate of absorption if you opt for the high-end stuff from a health and nutrition store.

Looking beyond the deficiency issue, sometimes there is a discrepancy between *minimum* and *optimal* micronutrient levels, particularly for exercisers. The recommended daily allowances (RDAs) for vitamins and minerals are set at the minimum amounts that appear to be required to avoid being sick, but those amounts aren't necessarily enough for a person to thrive.

Certain substances, one being creatine monohydrate, produce a significant effect when taken in doses that are impossible to obtain through food alone. Creatine is found in red meat, but you'd need to eat pounds of it every day to obtain what's considered to be a pharmaceutical dose of creatine. You can get by just fine without the extra creatine, but your friend who is following the same program and also supplementing with creatine will be leaner and stronger, with a higher metabolism and a lower bodyfat percentage.

Although creatine is the most noteworthy example, you may want to educate yourself on which supplements might be worth your while to use at times, particularly in cases where it's difficult, if not impossible, to obtain sufficient quantities of the substance simply by following a balanced diet. There is a good deal of controversy surrounding supplement recommendations, and you must be wary of distributors' claims since many are just looking to make a quick buck. However, not *everything* is snake oil, because the science is there to back up many of the claims that particular supplements are effective.

Some experts believe that vitamin C, for one, should be taken in megadoses while dieting. This antioxidant reduces free radicals and is known to aid in immunity and recovery. By maximizing your body's functioning, supplements like vitamin C can contribute to a higher metabolism.

Fish oil is another great supplement. If you live in the U.S. and don't supplement with essential fatty acids (EFAs), chances are you're deficient in them. When you have an EFA deficiency, you won't burn fat as efficiently and you'll have a tendency to lose lean body mass. The reason most people are deficient in EFAs is that, for the past 50 years or so, our food has been produced in a way that destroys naturally occurring EFAs in the diet. Unless you eat 4-6 oz. of the fattier fish (like salmon) at least twice per week or take two tablespoons of flaxseed or one tablespoon of flax oil every day, you are almost guaranteed to be deficient in the EFAs. Flaxseed isn't part of the mainstream American diet, and it can be risky to eat fish today due to the mercury content in seafood. I recommend 3-6 grams of fish oil taken daily for all the EFA supplementation you need.

Calcium is another biggie – this mineral promotes bone health, proper electrolyte balance, and fat loss. While calcium is important for everyone's bone health, women, and post-menopausal women in particular, are at a higher risk for osteoporosis. The recommendation for the number of dairy servings per day is higher for that group than for any other, yet post-menopausal women as group need fewer calories per day than everyone except the elderly. That means calcium supplements are especially helpful for post-menopausal women. Strong bones are one of the components of your lean body mass that helps keep metabolism high. You also need those bones to be strong so you can stay healthy and perform your workouts safely. Moreover, there have been a slew of studies done on calcium and fat loss in the past few years. It has been proven that calcium intake dictates rate of weight loss, even at the same calorie level (3). High-calcium groups lose 2-3 times the fat and 1/3 less muscle than low/moderate-calcium groups. This can mean the difference of losing 8 pounds of fat rather than just 3, while only losing 2 pounds of muscle instead of 3. In this example, the net weight loss would be 10 pounds in the high calcium group versus just 6 pounds in the low/moderate calcium group. Body composition is improved even more dramatically with a high-calcium intake. The low/moderate calcium group loses equal amounts of muscle and fat (and therefore, in spite of losing weight, stays at the same bodyfat percentage). On the other hand, the high-calcium group loses 8 pounds of fat and only 2 pounds of muscle! The low/moderate calcium group loses fat and muscle in a 1:1 ratio while dieting, but the high-calcium group loses fat at a 4:1 ratio to muscle. This means, for every 4 pounds of fat lost in the high-calcium group, only 1 pound of muscle is lost along with it. That's a *very* good ratio to achieve while dieting, since sometimes people lose even more muscle than fat when they're dieting.

Calcium makes a good case for the power of supplementation, since many people fall short of the recommended 3-4 servings of dairy products per day (900-1200 mg of calcium). It is true that you usually get better results consuming your nutrients from food rather than from supplements. However, a dietary supplement is far better than nothing and is invaluable in helping you fill the gaps in your diet.

Key 7: Get a good night's rest

6-9 hours of sleep (whichever amount leaves you feeling like you had a great night's rest and allows you to wake up without needing an alarm clock) sets the stage for an efficiently running metabolism. Chronic sleep loss affects the processing and storing of carbohydrates and the regulation of hormone secretion in the body. The effect can be so drastic that after just one week of poor sleep the changes in the body resemble the effects of advanced age and the early stages of diabetes (4). <u>Getting too little sleep also increases the secretion of cortisol, a stress hormone that eats away at muscle and bone tissue and increases the deposition of abdominal fat.</u> Yes, you can be so stressed out that you develop a gut! Maybe the phrase "beauty rest" isn't just a saying! If you have a roll of fat around the middle but don't have excess fat anywhere else, you can be pretty sure that cortisol is to blame.

So how does one get enough sleep? Well, the answer depends on the reason you might be a poor sleeper. Some people feel tired but purposefully stay up late and awaken early in an attempt to get more done. If you've been guilty of this, don't bother. You're harming your body too much, and it has been proven that sleep-deprived people are less productive during the day. Discipline yourself to stick to a set bedtime, and avoid watching TV or doing stressful work in bed.

Also, you can't expect to get a good night's sleep after drinking coffee or cola all day. Even if you are able to fall asleep initially, having caffeine in your system (this drug has a 4-hour half life, so yes, it is still in your system) makes for a less restful, less restorative sleep. You won't be able to hit the deep phases of sleep and stay there for the normal length of time if you've been using caffeine during the day. And the more caffeine you consume, the more harmful the effects. If you really love your coffee, 1 or 2 cups of joe in the morning shouldn't do much harm, although you *would* be healthier and would probably feel better in the long run without it. Consider switching to tea, which has less caffeine than coffee and contains other beneficial compounds that are good for your metabolism and your health. If you must have caffeine, have it as early in the day as possible. Keep in mind that quitting caffeine cold turkey usually results in headaches, lethargy, and temporary depression. It's recommended to wean off of caffeine over a period of 7-14 days.

If you're not sleeping well and these simple sleep habits don't help, you might need to see a sleep specialist. For more tips, turn to page 256 where you'll find the Better Sleep Council's "Ten Tips for Better Sleep." Just be sure that you don't put sleep on the back burner, because it's critically important on so many levels.

Well, there you have it: The seven foolproof tactics to raising your metabolism that you can start applying to your life – every one of them is guaranteed to affect your metabolism and your physique for the better. If you're following at least some of these principles and you're taking in a good amount of healthful calories, you should be able to lose unwanted bodyfat to the tune of 0.5-2.0 pounds per week, every week. You shouldn't have any problems maintaining the loss and you shouldn't hit any plateau that you can't overcome with a bit of tweaking to your program.

The "adequate calories" piece is an important part of all this – besides all the other reasons you need to eat regularly, eating is a thermogenic activity, meaning that it uses energy. In other words, eating calories burns calories! Some people are really gung-ho when they start dieting and do everything they can think of to raise their metabolism, and also try to eat as few calories as possible using tactics such as skipping meals, avoiding animal protein, avoiding all fat and/or carbs, and eating salad every day for lunch (if they even eat lunch at all). The body will go into an emergency state at that point to conserve calories and fat stores, because it picks up pretty quickly on the energy crisis. Having a too-large calorie deficit will sabotage your long-term weight loss goals because it will cause your metabolism to slow to a crawl. The ideal situation is for you to be eating about 500 calories less than you burn each day, resulting in steady weight loss without those rapid losses and even faster re-gains, and without finding yourself stalled on that dreaded plateau.

You can cut 500 calories out of your diet pretty easily if you pay attention to what you're consuming and are aware of the calorie content in common foods and beverages. For example, you can save 500 calories by passing on three cans of soda, three glasses of juice, or three glasses of wine, by saying no to that muffin or that handful of cookies, or by leaving four spoonfuls of food on your plate at breakfast, lunch, and dinner. You can also burn those 500 calories off through exercise – walking or running 5 miles will do it. Most people find that a combination of eating less and moving more is the easiest way for them to hit the 500-calorie deficit.

I know that the idea of incorporating these seven keys all at once might seem overwhelming. Don't worry, you can start with just one – I promise you, you will notice a difference. Usually addressing just one or two of the keys will leave you with the optimal calorie deficit, especially when you're just starting out. You can always decide to apply more of the principles in the future if you need to. You'd want to do this if you hit a plateau, or if you would like to be able to eat more than you have been and continue losing weight. Remember, think "progress" not "perfection." Every little bit helps. The very first thing you should do is adopt a resistance-training program if you haven't already. You'll be on the fast track to having a lean, toned body with a smartly designed weights routine.

III. Prep Work

Strategy 1: No Fear!

How to make a commitment to change

If you are studying this System, it's probably safe to assume that you want to change your health, your fitness, and your appearance for the better. To get started, there are only two things you need to do: make the decision to change, and the commitment to never look back. What separates those who are motivated to make the commitment from those who aren't? *The main reason you might not be determined to change a situation that has caused you pain is that you have a short-term memory.* Almost every behavior that has the potential to cause pain also offers up pleasure in the short-term. If you have a short-term memory, you'll be lured in by the short-term pleasure because you keep forgetting that the trade-off is long-term pain. Sometimes it takes hitting "rock-bottom" for a person to change, but hopefully you can make up your mind to change before it gets to that point. Ideally you will be able to use just the *thought* of future pain to help solidify your commitment to change *now*, without actually having to go through any more struggles.

You're going to need to use the most painful thoughts, feelings, and experiences you've had up until this point as a motivator to make your commitment to change. A painful motivator for you might have been the time someone made fun of the way you looked, or it could have been the time you avoided the beach so that you wouldn't be seen in a bathing suit. Maybe it was the time you found yourself gasping for breath climbing just two flights of stairs, or the time you hurt your back lifting something that really wasn't all that heavy.

Once you have committed to your decision to change, you will have passed the most difficult battle in this process. Upon solidifying your commitment your thoughts will be freed up, allowing you to become completely focused on your mission. Outside distractions will be minimized the more determined you become. You will make all of this easier on yourself by having the mindset, "no turning back." Rather than allow yourself to be intimidated by the process, make the choice to dive into it with no fear. This will give you the strength and the courage to change.

See, fear of change or of how you will cope robs energy from you that you simply can't afford to waste. Your thoughts have a good chance of becoming your reality, so be sure to keep them under your control. If something sidetracks you from your plan, use the slip to intensify your motivation, rather than as an excuse to throw in the towel. Make sure you take the time to pay attention to what has happened so you don't miss the opportunity to learn from your mistakes.

For instance, if you make the mistake of having something to eat that isn't on your diet plan, step back from any emotional reaction you might have for a moment so you can analyze the situation. Use the information you uncover to troubleshoot so that it's less likely to happen again. This lifestyle change you are undertaking is a *process*, not an event. The decision to commit to a path in the healthy direction *is* a one-time event, but you won't get the steps mapped out perfectly the first time you try. Any successful lifestyle change *has* to be an ongoing process of testing, applying, and adapting. What works for you today might not work next year, so you've got to stay on your toes.

Let's look at an instance where a mistake can be turned into a learning experience and an opportunity to adapt for the better. Here's the scenario:

> *You hosted a party for a friend. Of course there were leftovers, and we're not talking carrot sticks – it's leftover cake and cookies. You eat some of those cookies the next day, and the day after that. You say to yourself, "enough's enough!" but you end up having some cookies the third day, too.*

As simple as this story is, it speaks volumes about human psychology and behavior. What's going on here? Why did you eat that stuff? If you're like most people, you tend to eat more junk food when it's right there in front of you. Also, if you're like most people you don't normally go to the store just because you have a craving for cookies. Furthermore, you know that you don't go to other people's houses just to eat their cookies. It seems that the odds you'll eat cookies go up tremendously when you happen to have them in the house.

Upon reaching this realization, some people decide to challenge themselves to a "battle of willpower." They expect themselves to be able to keep cookies in the house without touching them. Well, maybe that *could* work, but why not make things easier and simpler by deciding to keep your house a "cookie-free zone?" What you have to understand is that you are *not* a weak person simply because you haven't been able to avoid eating those cookies. As a human being, your body is wired to crave calorie-dense foods full of fat and sugar. These foods are the ones most readily converted into bodyfat, which is something your body is wired to do for survival in case there's a time of shortage.

Despite your best intentions, odds are you'll end up eating

things you wish you hadn't if you're surrounded by them all the time. The fact that you want them so badly when they are within reach is a testament to your genetic qualities more than anything else. See, almost all the families that are alive today are the ones who were "better" than the rest at survival. The ones on the earth today for the most part come from hardy stock. Without that strong survival instinct, your ancestors probably would have died out during difficult times.

If this makes sense to you and you're willing to try other solutions besides relying on "willpower," the next step should be obvious: Don't keep "trigger" foods in the house! Even if those foods end up on your countertop for whatever reason, you still have options. Try putting the food in the freezer until someone will take it from you, or donate it to a food pantry. Even if you end up throwing the food in the trash, it would have been "wasted" anyway if you ate it against your will, since all you'd be left with is excess weight on your body.

I know that this idea of not keeping the food at home sounds simplistic, but it's amazing how many people refuse to "get" it and continue to sabotage themselves. Maybe it would be great if you had willpower made of steel and weren't tempted when that fattening stuff was sitting right there in the kitchen. However, the reality is that it's natural to be tempted by it, so why test yourself over and over and make it so difficult? Why have the tempting foods so easily accessible? The smartest thing to do, if impulse eating is a problem for you, is to use your willpower where it's better served and more useful: *When you're in the store, use it to avoid buying junk food in the first place, or use it to avoid taking the stuff home when it's offered to you.*

This is a less arduous task and is less "dangerous" than testing yourself once you actually have the fattening foods lying around at home. If you're like most people, your guard will be lowered in your own home, not to mention the fact that you'll probably have more downtime at home with the kitchen at easy access. Downtime at home is a time when you're likely to seek comfort (which some people find through eating). It's also the time when you're most susceptible to making an impulse decision, since your guard will be let down when you're relaxing at home.

Downtime is not the only thing that can be damaging for your waistline, however. Stress can be just as harmful. Stress makes some people eat more, while it causes others lose their appetite. Sometimes the motivation to seek comfort in certain foods comes from the need to escape a myriad of emotions. Any emotion, whether it's positive or negative, can trigger you to indulge in junk food or extra-large portions.

Hopefully this example of how you can take control at home will inspire you to think of other ways you can manipulate your environment to make your life easier. Once you've developed the capacity to separate your emotional needs from food, you will have much more control over your eating. The easiest place to start is at home, since you will have more control over your environment there. Once you develop more control over your eating in that situation, you will feel empowered to tackle obstacles in the outside world. If you've got things under control on the home front, you won't have to worry about that area too much anymore and should be more confident that you can handle any temptation you may encounter in the outside world.

With all this talk about handling temptation and avoiding junk food, you might be wondering if it's okay to treat yourself by having a food you really like that isn't the healthiest or most diet-friendly. You'll be happy to know that I am a firm believer in enjoying a treat once in a while. The difference between "giving in" and treating yourself is that, once you have the ability to control what you're eating, *it will be your choice* to have it. Therefore, the treat will be a source of pleasure (rather than a source of pain because you feel bad for "giving in"). It will be a source of pleasure to indulge yourself once you have control because you'll know you can *choose* whether or not to have it. Plus, when you're in control, you will find it much easier to stop at one small serving and feel satisfied.

If you live by yourself, all the advice I've given so far should work just fine. However, things will be more complicated if you live with other people who might not be willing to give up keeping some junk food around.

If this is the case for you, the first thing you'll need to do is clearly separate in your mind which foods are for you and which foods are for your roommate, your kids or your significant other. If you fail to do this, you might find yourself picking from your kids' plates after dinner or eating their snacks when they don't finish them. You might find yourself eating your husband's potato chips or your wife's Ben and Jerry's. Many times, you're eating this stuff simply because it's around, not because you really want it. If you can draw a clear line between what you are and are not going to eat, you can make a rule for yourself that will take away the need to make a new decision every day about whether or not you'll eat the junk.

You can certainly still treat yourself here and there, but you don't want to be eating junk food just because it's there. You want to save your indulgences for times when you *really* have a craving, and at those times should have what you want most, not just what happens to be around. You can literally start *ignoring* certain foods if you make the clear-cut decision that you simply don't eat them. I'm sure that there are some foods you've already ruled out in your mind that simply don't pose a problem for you anymore. Even if you've ruled out a food because you don't like it, it doesn't matter – you still have proven that it's possible for you to rule out certain foods.

For example, let's say that you read an article in a magazine about the ten most fattening foods you can order at a fast-food restaurant. Let's say hypothetically that a bacon double-cheeseburger was on that list, and it contains 1,100 calories and 65 grams of fat (that number is not far off, but will vary a bit depending on where you order the sandwich). Right then and there, upon reading that information you might have decided, "I will never eat another bacon double-cheeseburger again. It's not worth it." Most likely, you weren't haunted by thoughts of that sandwich (don't laugh – people really do feel "haunted" by intense cravings) because *it simply wasn't an option for you anymore*. By making it a point to mentally categorize foods, you can make following your diet plan much, much easier. To understand just how powerful this technique can be, think back to a time when you used to frequent a particular store or restaurant for a food that wasn't the healthiest thing you could be eating. When you went there all the time, didn't it seem like you were on automatic pilot? Wasn't it hard to say no? If you stopped going there for whatever reason, I bet you hardly think about the place and that food anymore. I know this has happened to me many times.

If you try to create rules for yourself with food and are still struggling with having your family's food around at home, I recommend assigning a "designated shelf" for the food that you will commit to staying away from. In the worst-case scenario where the temptation still proves to be too much, ask your family to keep the food in their bedrooms or otherwise hidden from you. This might seem silly or over-the-top, but it definitely works. Some people have a *really* difficult time when they are told they can't have something, so there is a chance that you might have to resort to drastic measures if you're serious about staying away from it. An added bonus is that, even if you *do* manage to stumble across the hidden food, you will probably be too embarrassed to eat any, lest the owner of the food take notice!

Now, I'd like to say a few words regarding slips off your diet plan: If this happens, it just doesn't make sense to throw in the towel. Instead, think about the fact that you still have the same goal and are still just as determined to reach it. After a slip you'll be armed with a new tool in your pocket, which is the experience of having a slip and figuring out what went wrong. Having gone through the experience and analyzed it, you're less likely to allow the same mistake to happen again. After you've analyzed what happened, your game plan will be that much stronger. This is a very different attitude and approach from giving up and throwing in the towel after a slip. Giving up is the easiest thing to do in the short-term, but your problem will *not* have gone away. In the long run, learning from your mistake and moving forward will serve you so much better. You'll be much happier and a lot more successful, too.

What if your problem with junk food isn't really at home, but you find yourself overindulging when you're out and about at parties or in restaurants? In this case, you can take control of your environment mentally if not physically. You need to decide before the event what you would like to do. If you've been following a healthy diet and feel that it's time for a little bit of planned indulgence, decide to follow the "80/20 Rule" and take small portions of the foods you crave. For more information on the 80/20 Rule, see Reference B in the back of the book.

Maybe on a particular day you'd rather stick to your usual way of eating even though you're going out. You can mentally "take control of your environment" just like you can physically take control over which foods you keep at home. Just make sure you decide what you will do before temptation strikes. If you're planning to stick to eating healthy, you need to mentally remove the option to have the junk. You'll be surprised how much easier it feels to say no when you commit to what you want to do beforehand. If any thoughts about changing your mind start to creep into your head, *the key is to not even allow yourself to entertain the option of changing your mind.* You can tell yourself that you'll have the option to indulge next time if you choose, but for today you're sticking to your decision. Being in control of what you do really can be that simple. See Reference B for tips on how to eat healthy in all types of restaurants, including fast-food places.

You'll want to experiment with various foods and recipes to find things you really enjoy that also happen to be healthy. Also, it will behoove you to find ways to treat yourself that don't involve food. There are plenty of options, and you'll get a chance to brainstorm some of them in one of the assignments for this Strategy.

No Fear! assignment

1.   Forming a mission statement is common practice for most companies and organizations. The mission statement helps to align everyone's behavior toward a common goal.

Brainstorm some ideas for a personal "mission statement." Your "mission statement" will help you align your thoughts and behaviors toward your desired outcome. I want you to write your mission statement as if you have already accomplished the outcome. This means it will end up looking more like a "mission accomplished statement." One example of a "mission accomplished statement" is, "I eat 3 nutritious meals and 2 snacks every day, and follow the 80/20 Rule with food." Another example of a "mission accomplished statement" is, "I do my weights routine and my cardio 3 times per week for 8 weeks at a time, and then I take one week off." Once you settle on one or two "mission accomplished statements," post them someplace where you can see them every day.

2.   Start a 30-day commitment journal in a blank notebook. Write your "mission accomplished statement" in big letters on the first page. Across the top of the next three pages write, "How I used to be." Divide each of those pages into two columns. In the first column, list the things you used to do that got you nothing but poor results. Across the page from each entry, list the painful consequences you experienced and/or the painful consequences that could be soon to come if you continue with your old ways. After you're finished coming up with as many examples as you can, keep these pages held together with a paperclip. Only reference them if you find yourself repeating some of your old behaviors, simply to remind yourself what you should expect as a result. Occasionally you may have a need to remind yourself what doing those things got you before. Otherwise, there is no need to stay in the negative, and no sense in filling your brain with "don'ts." Your mind will remain fixated on the words and ideas that run through your head, which means that you risk harming yourself if you ruminate about things that have gone wrong in the past. The only time it might be beneficial to think about the pain you experienced is if you find yourself tempted to stray from your commitment to change. If you have truly committed to making a change, this shouldn't happen. However, you are only human and you might find yourself feeling tempted at times, particularly during the first two weeks of your

commitment. Sometimes just the act of changing, even if it's not such a bad change, can be tough and you might rebel since it's more comforting to continue doing what is familiar. If you find yourself struggling to maintain your commitment, you might want to keep a reminder of the pain you experienced with you at all times to help fight off that "short-term memory" syndrome. I know people who keep a picture of themselves looking particularly out-of-shape in their day-planner or on their mirror as a constant reminder of the pain they experienced. If doing something like this helps you, then by all means do it. Just be careful not to spend too much time tossing around negative thoughts.

3.   Come up with a list of foods that never seem to tempt you – list them on the next blank page of your notebook. Be sure to include *all* the foods that don't tempt you – it doesn't matter what the reason is. Some of the foods that you'll put on your list don't tempt you simply because you don't like them. Others don't tempt you because you just never eat them, or because you decided to stop eating them at one point and haven't thought twice about it since.

For example, my list of foods that never seem to tempt me includes pork, sausage, squash, and anything made with garlic (I don't like them). It also includes hamburgers, fried food, and potato chips (I like them somewhat, but I stopped eating them awhile ago and don't miss them when I don't have them.). My list further includes full-fat ice cream, sugary cereal, and muffins. Although I like these foods, I don't care to have them even as treats because there are plenty of other treats that are less fattening or that I enjoy more. Therefore, for me these foods aren't "worth" going off my diet plan.

See how many foods you can come up with for your list. You might surprise yourself with how many things you are able to avoid pretty effortlessly already. Work on expanding your list in the future so that you can improve your diet and make healthy eating easier on yourself.

4.   Write "troubleshooting" across the top of the next three blank pages of your notebook. Divide each of these pages into two columns. I would like you to come back to these pages and fill in this chart during your 30-day commitment as you strive to live your "mission accomplished statement." If you make a mistake and deviate from your plan, write the mistake in the first column, and across the page in the next column write the changes you'll make in

order to prevent it from happening again. For example, let's say that you skip a workout because you would rather watch a certain program on TV. Your troubleshoot might be, "next time I will tape the program and only allow myself to watch it once I've completed my workout."

5. Lots of assignments for this chapter! On the next blank page in your notebook, come up with a list of pleasurable activities other than eating junk food. Eating fattening foods seems to be one of the quickest and easiest solutions we use to give ourselves pleasure, especially in today's society. However, if you think hard you can probably come up with many other things that might even be more enjoyable for you that don't have negative consequences like being overweight and unhealthy. Refer back to this list if you find yourself in need of some ideas on how to indulge yourself, and copy some of your favorites into your day planner so you'll have your options at easy access. This should help you avoid acting on your first pleasure-seeking impulse, which might be to overeat. Remember, overeating is instinctive for many people. This doesn't have to pose a problem as long as you're aware of it and you develop the capacity to control that initial impulse. In order to be successful at controlling your initial impulse to overeat, it's important that you feed your body enough calories and you eat every few hours. If you do those things, you shouldn't ever feel super-hungry and your body won't perceive the threat of malnutrition. This makes it much easier both physically and psychologically to bypass your initial impulse to overeat or have junk food.

Strategy 2: Stop Procrastinating

How to increase your productivity and decrease your level of stress

Did you complete the assignment for the "No Fear!" Strategy? If you did, that's great – you're right on track for making a lasting change. If you didn't – what are you waiting for? This System is meant to be an interactive resource. It won't help you nearly as much if you just read through it without seeing how the information fits into your life via the assignments. Unless you've been doing pretty well with your health and fitness already and are just skimming the book for additional tips, please take the time to complete the assignments for each Strategy before you move on to read about another topic. Not only will completing the assignments help you to remember the Strategy much better, but doing them will also help guide you in starting to apply what you've learned to your life. The assignments help bridge the gap between theory and application. They will make the information in the Strategies ten times more valuable to you and are the most important part of this program. Did you know that over 95% of self-help books never get acted upon? Don't be part of that statistic! I want you to succeed, and I would love to receive feedback on how the program works for you. If you've been working out and eating well prior to getting your hands on this System, you may not have a need to do all the assignments. If that's the case for you, just pick and choose the ones that look to be more helpful, but be sure to complete them before moving on. Okay, I'll step off my soapbox now! Moving on...

Procrastinating has to be one of the most useless actions (or, more accurately, lack of action) there is. It's important that you realize procrastination is completely different from relaxation. Everyone needs rest and relaxation built into his schedule. Downtime is very important for a person's health and happiness. When stress levels rise too high, many hormones in your body are adversely affected. Just one of the changes associated with a state of chronically high stress is increased bodyfat storage, in particular the accumulation of fat in the abdominal region. As we all know, excess abdominal fat has negative implications for appearance and for health.

There is a dark side to procrastination beyond the effects on your physique and your physical health, however. When you procrastinate, it is incredibly harmful because not only are you getting nothing accomplished, you aren't completely relaxing either because in the back of your mind you are thinking about what you *should* be doing. This means you lose out on your relaxation time too, since you're spending so much time procrastinating. If you find yourself procrastinating on a regular basis, you're going to need to formally schedule all the tasks you'd like to complete each day, even the little things.

One of the reasons that personal training in fitness is becoming increasingly popular is that people tend to respect the time reserved for their workout if they have a scheduled appointment. By committing another person's time as well as your money to the workout, you are much less likely to skip. What you've done by setting an appointment is you've increased the level of pain you will experience if you blow it off. Some of my clients use a trainer mainly for this reason – they know they'd be at risk to skip their workout otherwise. If you want the accountability but don't want to use a trainer for every workout, consider meeting with a workout partner every time you train. I also have some clients who email me when they complete their workouts. Just something as simple as keeping your own workout log can help, too. The reward for jumping right in and getting everything done is that you will have more time to rest and relax at the end of the day, free of stress and guilt.

It's a given that each day is going to pass no matter what. *The only way you can fail is if you do nothing.* You, and only you, decide whether you get closer to or further from your goal. This is a decision that no coach, mentor, or trainer can make for you. If you do nothing you will simply fall further and further away from your goal of having a healthy, fit body. The reason you go backwards if you do nothing is that your body won't even stay at status quo if you don't exercise it. As you age, you experience a loss of body tone *unless you exercise consistently.* On the other hand, if you exercise regularly, your body usually won't look its age. People will tend to guess you to be younger and younger than you really are the longer you've been exercising consistently.

Bodies require ongoing maintenance and care. The good news is if you spend about three hours a week on your physical fitness, you will reap all the rewards that come with having a fit body. Even by spending just 30 focused minutes a week, you can experience tremendous benefit (see Reference C, "Just How Much Time is Required to Experience the Benefits of Exercise?") On the other hand, if you neglect your body's need for physical activity, you *will* suffer the consequences – if not now, then surely later. Any step in the right direction, which includes reading this System, is to be commended. There is no perfect time, perfect plan, or perfect effort. Make strides in the right direction at your own pace and you *will* reap the benefits.

After about 30 days of consistency, your new outlook and behaviors will have become habit and procrastination will be much less of an issue. It will start feeling normal and natural for you to complete your workouts and practice healthy eating. I know it's a cliché, but every journey really does begin with one step. Every proud owner of a tight, fit body started out with that same step. Get on it now – don't let any more time pass you by!

Stop Procrastinating assignment

1. Make a list of excuses you might come up with to eat poorly or miss a workout on the next two pages in your notebook.

2. On the following page, make two columns. Group the excuses you came up with into two categories: "Legitimate excuses" and "Illegitimate excuses." Make sure you give some thought as to which group your excuse belongs in, because you will have to stick to your choice if you find yourself trying to use the excuse one of these days. In the future, if you find yourself with a "reason" to miss a workout, you can check to see if your excuse is a valid one in your eyes. For example, let's say that you group "I have a fever" as a legitimate excuse and "I am behind on household chores" as an illegitimate excuse. If you find yourself trying to use a legitimate excuse not to work out in the future, you still need to get that workout in at some point during your week, but you may permit yourself to reschedule it. If you try to use one of your illegitimate excuses, you are going to need to reassess whether having a fit, healthy body is important to you or not. If you decide that it is, your illegitimate excuse just won't fly.

Make sure you tackle your excuses for eating poorly too. Examples include, "It's a holiday and I'm going to indulge" and, "I'm too tired to make anything tonight, so I think I'll order pizza." Which excuses will be legitimate and which will be illegitimate?

A surefire way to make sure all your workouts get done is to schedule them ahead of time. If you have to miss one due to a legitimate excuse, you may permit yourself to make it up at a future time or date. Strive to maintain your commitment to a certain number of workouts per week or month and a certain level of healthy eating, barring the most extenuating of circumstances.

If for some reason you miss too much time to make up the workouts, just resume your schedule as normal. In the big picture, as long as you get yourself back on track, missed workouts won't be a big deal. The ultimate key to fitness is to maintain as much consistency as possible over the long run. The reason I encourage trying to make up missed workouts is so that you won't feel like you can avoid working out by putting it off. Oftentimes you'll find that you *can* fit your workout in after all if you just get creative, since it seems like even more of a pain to figure out how you can fit it in later on.

It's amazing how drastically your hierarchy of priorities can change when you create a different set of rules for yourself. Your rules should be based on what you want most in life. I have no interest in *forcing* you to do your workouts and eat right, nor should you have to force yourself. You just need to understand that certain goals are going to require certain actions to get you there. There is no "free lunch." If you really do want that great body, you need to do the work to get it. The rules you have for maintaining your health and fitness are simply the vehicles that allow you to get what you want out of life. Workouts and healthy meals are not to be resented. If it really seems *that* bad, it probably won't be worth it to you. However, if you decide that you really *do* want to tone up, get healthier, and feel better, you need to resign yourself to the fact that it's going to require some effort.

Keep in mind, too, that you will have rest days built into your schedule, and you'll get to enjoy "vacations" from dieting and exercising. These periods of downtime are actually an important part of your overall progress. The "80/20 Rule" in Reference B discusses "cheat" days and "cheat" meals, and there is an entire Strategy devoted to rest (Strategy 29). The danger I'm addressing here and now is missing scheduled workouts. While missing one workout might not seem like much, missing a workout is the number-one precursor to a person giving up on a program. One missed session turns into two, two into three, and so on. Even if you don't allow yourself to slide downhill, you still don't want to miss any workouts. You'll only be falling behind in your journey toward your ultimate goal, and perhaps more importantly, you'll stop taking your goals so seriously. This just isn't the right attitude to have when you claim to be determined to achieve something.

Strategy 3: Talking "up"

How to use positive self-talk to promote success

Everything will become easier for you once you reach the understanding that you create your own reality. You will find that more positive things come into your life almost effortlessly when you utilize positive self-talk. The thoughts and images that fill your mind include both what's real and what's imaginary, and your mind can't tell the difference – all it knows are the thoughts and images that are in your head. You can use this lack of differentiation between the real and the imaginary to your advantage. To capitalize on this phenomenon, always be thinking about what you *want* to have happen. Your mind will interpret this thought as if it's already come true.

Your mind will focus most on the concepts that dominate your thoughts. Do you see, then, why it's better to think, "I am getting stronger every day" rather than, "I am very weak?" Your mind will focus on the *main idea* of a thought (for the previous example, the main idea is "stronger every day" and "very weak," respectively). That's one reason why it's better to think positive thoughts. Also, realize that your mind tends to focus on the main idea so intensely that it sometimes misses qualifier words like "don't." Therefore, it's better to think "I workout 3 times a week" than it is to think, "I don't skip my workouts." Your brain will tend to focus on the main idea, which is "workout 3 times a week" or "skip my workouts" in that example. Which would you rather have happen?

If you need proof of just how powerful your mind can be, think back to a time when you felt petrified of something that wasn't actually right there in front of you at the moment. When you were a child, were you ever afraid of monsters that you imagined might be there, even though you couldn't see them at the time? Your brain sent signals to your body that there was something to be afraid of, in spite of the fact that you couldn't actually see anything amiss. What about a time when you were walking alone in an unfamiliar place? Did you ever feel afraid even though there was no sign of immediate danger? If this has happened to you, your brain perceived the threat that you imagined as reality, and this became manifest in your body. In this type of situation, your breathing might have become shallow, your heart might have started beating faster, and you might have developed goose bumps, all because of something you imagined!

The moral of the story is to keep your thoughts positive, rather than let your mind focus on what you *shouldn't* do. Better yet, create your own reality and turn an "I should do" into an "I do." You greatly improve your chances for success when you maintain a positive mindset. You can actually psyche yourself out when you focus on the negative by thinking about all the bad things that *could* happen.

I know from participating in competitive gymnastics that this can happen very easily. I remember certain instances when I told myself "I can't" and, sure enough, it came true. Many times it took my coach telling me he believed in me before I'd start planting those positive ideas into my head. I didn't learn every move I wanted to in my career, but the tougher ones that I learned came as a result of positive thinking. This example also reinforces a message from the "No Fear!" Strategy. Sometimes you get the best results when you place blind faith in a mentor who knows what's best for you, even if what that mentor recommends feels uncomfortable or unnatural at first.

It might feel funny to start telling yourself, "I am losing weight every day" if you know it's not true yet. Keep at it anyway, because this type of self-talk will unleash mental power that you might not even know you had. Your experience will be similar to what I went through when I had the ability to do a gymnastics skill but I just wasn't confident enough until my coach insisted that I could. You have so much untapped power inside, and using these techniques will help you to release it. You can develop a ton of confidence in yourself simply by using positive self-talk. This confidence will give you the strength to maximize your abilities, enabling you to put your best effort forth in everything you do.

Talking "up" assignment

1. On the next page in your notebook, I'd like you to list some positive phrases relating to your goals. Make sure they're stated in the affirmative. For example:
    a. "I choose fruit when I want a sweet."
    b. "I commit to working out for at least 10 minutes no matter what."
    (Many times you will feel a surge of energy and motivation and want to continue! But even if you don't, at least you did *something*. You got closer to your goal).
    c. "I take my multivitamin every morning with breakfast."
    (Or even, "I eat breakfast." You know who you are!)

2. Refer to this page often. You might get some ideas for your goals by referring back to section II of this book, "The 7 Keys to Raising Your Metabolism for Life." Come up with your own ideas that are best suited to your needs, in particular ones that can help you reverse the poisonous effects of negative thinking.

    To expand your list, consider any statements that you find running though your head, even if they are negative. Give the negative ones a positive spin and write it down. For instance, if you find yourself thinking, "I can't seem to stay away from those cookies – I'm getting so fat!" turn that thought into, "I reach for fruits, vegetables, and yogurt when I need a snack. I am getting thinner every day." I know that might sound corny to you, but you will thank me for the suggestion when you achieve all your goals.

    Repetition is the only way you're going to cement these thoughts into your head. You might want to transfer the positive statements from your notebook onto index cards so you'll have them at easy access. Keep the cards in a handy place so you can flip through them when you have a minute. At the very least, keep them by your bed and go through them each night before going to sleep. They will stick in your memory better when you read them at that time. Or, jot them down in your day planner so that every time you open it you can glance at them. This will help to reinforce your positive mindset.

Strategy 4: You are the Feature Presentation

How to visualize success

You will find it immensely helpful not only to write your goals down and rehearse empowering statements, but also to visualize yourself completing the steps that will be part of the process. To try visualization, your first inclination might be to view yourself as if you're watching a movie of your life. However, this is not the most effective method of visualization if your purpose is to increase your chances of making your vision a reality. A more effective technique is to visualize yourself going through each experience *as it would look through your own eyes*. In other words, you want to "view" the scene as it would appear through your own eyes rather than by "witnessing" the scene by watching your figure from another person's perspective.

Make sure to include *all* the necessary steps, even the little ones that may seem obvious or unimportant. Also, I'd like you to use all of your senses in this "visualization," not just the sense of sight. The term "visualization" is the recognized term used to describe this process of imagining yourself doing something, so I'll continue to use it even though you need to use all your senses for this process to be most effective.

For instance, if one of your goals is to be able to jog for a cardio workout, "visualize" yourself changing into athletic clothes, putting on your socks and shoes, going out the front door, and breaking into a trot – all as it would look through your own eyes. If it is springtime, imagine how the fresh, crisp air smells. Imagine the sensation of your mouth starting to dry and the relief you get from taking a sip of water. Imagine the feel of your foot in your sneakers landing on the pavement with a thud and the flex of your calf muscle as you push off the ground through your toes. Finally, imagine the feeling of satisfaction that washes over you as you finish the run. I left out quite a few details in this scene – try it for yourself and see how detailed you can make your visualization!

During my career as a competitive gymnast, I found that my performance improved tremendously when I used visualization. I used to visualize myself doing a difficult move correctly before I'd actually make the attempt. Sometimes I'd visualize a famous gymnast doing the move and that would help too. The main reason visualizing a pro helped was because they made it look easy, and that made the move seem less intimidating. You might choose to visualize someone you admire doing what you would like to be able to do yourself. I still believe, however, that the most powerful type of visualization is to visualize yourself, because that's the best way to increase your confidence. Personally, I use both types.

You have so many capabilities that you just haven't learned to tap into yet. Visualization helps bridge the gap between what you *want* to do and what you *are actually capable of* once you break through any mental barriers that might be holding you back. The toughest barrier to get through is the lack of belief that you can do it. Visualization "tricks" your brain into thinking you are already doing whatever it is you wish to achieve. This belief is what will allow you to reach your full potential. Having unshakable belief can only help as you work to achieve your goals.

Your life is the Feature Presentation assignment

1. In your notebook, list several actions you plan to take at some point on the way to achieving your goals. Before you go to sleep or during a spare moment in your day, pick one action to visualize. For instance, let's assume that one of your actions will be doing cardio at the gym. Try to visualize this process. Make sure you start your visualization from the very beginning. In this case, the script would include all the steps involved in getting dressed for the gym, leaving your house, and getting in the car – all the way up to the actual workout and the completion of the workout, as well as how you feel afterward. Take at least five minutes to go through the entire scenario in your head. As long your visualization is vivid enough, your mind won't be able to differentiate whether your visualization is real or imaginary. Be sure to utilize all the senses in your visualization, such as any sounds, smells, and sensations you might experience. Visualization works wonders because the more you practice success, the easier and more natural it becomes!

2. Get into the habit of visualizing yourself doing something new before you actually try it. Try starting your visualization a few days before you plan to try the real thing. If you visualize beforehand, you'll "psyche yourself up" for the day when you make it a reality.

Strategy 5: Applying discipline and creating S.M.A.R.T. Goals

How goal-mapping ensures your success

To increase the odds you'll achieve everything you want to do, you need to form highly specific goals. Then you need to break down each goal into a series of steps that will pave the way to your desired result. You'll increase your odds of success when you separate and identify each individual action that will be required to achieve an end result. This System should give you a good idea of what you can realistically set out to achieve with your health, your fitness, and your body shape.

You'll need to decide on a realistic time frame during which you'd like to achieve your goals. This will require a careful review of your history, and perhaps some additional research on your part or a consultation with a health and fitness expert. You might want to consult with your general physician as well. Just keep in mind that most medical doctors focus on pathology of the body and are not specifically trained to help an already healthy person strive for optimal health. A wellness consultant (the category that a health-oriented personal trainer fits into) is in business to help people thrive, which is the step beyond simply being free of illness. A typical medical school curriculum involves years of studying infection, cancer, chronic illness, and other forms of disease, but includes only a couple of lectures on proper nutrition. Moreover, doctors don't usually have the time to keep up-to-date on the latest developments in the health and fitness field. They simply have too many other things to worry about related to their principal task, which is to rid people of illness. Ideally, doctors would be able to provide specific advice on how to attain optimal health, but the reality is that their main focus lies elsewhere.

When forming your goals, you need to make sure that what you set out to do is realistically attainable for you. Also, make sure that you have an appropriate time frame in mind. For example, let's consider the proposed goal of losing 20 pounds in two months. The first question you need to ask is if it's *possible* for you to lose 20 pounds in a healthy manner. If so, is it possible to lose the weight in a healthy manner in two months' time? For some people, this rate of weight loss *is* realistic, healthy, and safe, but for the vast majority it *is not*, particularly if you want those lost pounds to come from bodyfat. Losing 20 pounds isn't so impressive if it comes from a loss of muscle or if it just represents a temporary reduction in water weight.

Anyone can lose a significant amount of water weight pretty quickly – all you need to do to drop water is take over-the-counter diuretics and cut back on sodium and carbohydrates for a couple of days. Losing bodyfat is what really matters, and each pound is a real victory. Each pound of bodyfat you lose represents about 3,500 calories burned and not replaced with calories from food. You can achieve that through applying the 7 Keys to raising metabolism, including regular exercise and maintaining a balanced diet.

Although you don't need to do everything perfectly to lose weight, if anything is *really* amiss in your overall program, it could sabotage your weight loss to the point that you won't lose a thing. In other words, if you do all the things that are important for weight loss fairly well (but not perfectly) you're much more likely to be successful than if you do most things perfectly but have one factor that is completely off. In other words, you'll be better off if you score "8s" across the board on all the 7 Keys than you'll be if you score six "10s" and one "2." I've seen people who can lose all the weight they want by making just one change, such as adding a couple of cardio sessions per week, but for the most part that's because cardio was the missing link for them and they had already been doing most of the other "7 Keys." As long as you don't have a glaring weakness in a certain area, small changes can result in big weight loss. It can just as easily go haywire, though.

For example, let's say that you decide to add five cardio workouts per week to your exercise routine, each workout consisting of a three-mile jog. Each of these five days you'll burn an extra 300 calories, meaning you'll have burned an extra 1500 over the five days. If on a whim you decide to have a small meat-lovers pizza as a late night snack, you effectively negated all that cardio with the pizza! That's what makes weight loss hard at times – there are many factors that will affect your results, and falling short in just one particular area can grind your weight-loss progress to a halt, even if you're doing everything else right. Don't make the mistake of focusing solely on weight loss: You'll still increase your fitness level when you work out, regardless of your diet – exercise is always worthwhile. If you're really going after weight loss, however, be sure to focus on diet and lifestyle in addition to exercise, because working out alone might not do it.

By being conscious of what you need to do to succeed, nothing that could sabotage your progress should slip by your radar. By making sure your goals are S.M.A.R.T. and by making sure that you have them mapped out so they lead to your final desired result, you should have no problem achieving anything you want in life.

Apply discipline assignment

1.   Check to see if your goals are S.M.A.R.T. (5). If not, modify them until they fit the criteria.

Source: Paul J. Meyer's "Attitude Is Everything."
http://www.topachievement.com/smart.html

Creating S.M.A.R.T. Goals

Specific
Measurable
Attainable
Realistic
Tangible

Specific. A specific goal (rather than a vague or general goal) has a much greater chance of being accomplished.

To set a specific goal, you must ask and answer the six "W" questions:

*Who: Who is involved?
*What: What do I want to accomplish?
*Where: Identify a location.
*When: Establish a time frame.
*Which: Identify requirements and constraints.
*Why: Specific reasons, purpose or benefits of accomplishing the goal.

For example, "get in shape" is a general goal. A specific goal would sound more like, "Complete my full-body weights routine that my trainer designed for me Monday, Wednesday and Friday this week." The specific goal has clear criteria, meaning that it's easy to say whether or not the goal was met.

Measurable. Establish concrete criteria for measuring progress toward the attainment of each goal you set. When you measure your progress, you are more likely to stay on track and reach your target dates for your short-term goals. This means you'll get to experience the sense of achievement that will inspire you to continue the effort required to reach your long-term goal.

To determine if your goal is measurable, ask questions such as:

*How much?
*How many?
*How will I know when it is accomplished?

For example, the goal "Lose four pounds of bodyfat this month" is a measurable one, whereas the goal, "I'd like to tone up" is not.

Attainable. When you identify goals that are important to you, you will become more motivated to figure out ways to make them come true. Only then will you develop the attitudes, abilities, skills, and financial capacity necessary to reach them. Once you feel really motivated, for the first time you'll start to see previously overlooked opportunities to bring yourself closer to the achievement of your goals.

You can attain almost any goal you set when you choose your steps wisely and establish a plan and a time frame that allows you to carry out those steps. Goals that may have seemed far away and out of reach eventually get closer and become attainable, not because your goals shrink, but because *you* grow and expand to match them. When you list your goals on paper, you build your self-image. You see yourself as worthy of these goals, and you start developing the traits and personality that enable you to accomplish them.

I know quite a few people who maintain an illusive goal in their head. A common one I hear as a trainer is, "I want to tone up." If a person is 50 pounds overweight, looking "toned up" seems far, far away. However, if he could break down that long-term goal into steps, such as losing five pounds at a time, the goal becomes attainable as long as you tackle the steps systematically. If your long-term goal is overwhelming to think about, it is easy to give up and just do nothing. However, once you take the time to break it down into mini-goals and you know the specific steps that are necessary to achieve them, you will realize that you *do* have what it takes to get to your long-term goal.

Realistic. To be realistic, a goal must represent an objective toward which you are both *willing* and *able* to work. Keep in mind that you can have a lofty goal that's still realistic – you are the only one who can decide just how high your goal should be.

While you need to make sure your goal is realistic, it is important that every goal represent substantial progress. A high goal oftentimes feels easier to reach than a low one because a low goal exerts low motivational force. With a low goal, you won't experience the adrenaline surge that happens when you're faced with a formidable challenge. Some of the hardest jobs you've ever tackled may actually have seemed easy simply because they were a labor of love, or because they caused you to push yourself and you found that exciting. However, if a goal is so high that it's unrealistic, you will lose your momentum quickly.

To test whether your goal is realistic, ask yourself if you truly *believe* that it can be accomplished. Another way to determine if your goal is realistic is to think about whether you have accomplished anything that was just as difficult in the past. You might also ask yourself what conditions would have to exist to accomplish the goal, and if it is possible for you to create that environment at this time.

For instance, it's not realistic for someone who has never tried running and gets winded climbing stairs to set the goal of running a 5-minute mile by next month. That person may be able to run a mile if he trains for it, however, and might even be able to break an 8-minute mile by the next month or two. On the other hand, a realistic goal for a world champion in the mile run is going to be a lot different. A realistic goal for a world champion might be improving his time from 3:52 to 3:49 by the next year. As you can see, realistic goals will be highly individualized, relative to abilities and past accomplishments. Also, beginners will make bigger jumps in progress than advanced exercisers.

Tangible - A goal is tangible when you can experience it with one of the senses, whether it's the sense of touch, taste, smell, sight or sound. When your goal is tangible, or when you tie a tangible goal to an intangible goal, you have a better chance of it being specific and measurable and therefore attainable.

Intangible goals are your goals for the internal changes required to reach the tangible goals you've set. They are the character traits and the behavior patterns you must develop that will pave the way to success. Since intangible goals are vital for improving your effectiveness, be sure to come up with *tangible* ways you can measure them.

For instance, if you have the intangible goal of being a more disciplined person, commit to a workout schedule for one month, and check back at the end of the month to see how you did.

2. Choose a long-term goal you'd like to tackle first, and start brainstorming steps that will lead to its attainment. For example, if your long-term goal is "lose 10 pounds by the New Year" and today it's November 1, you need to start by naming the steps that will put you on the path toward achieving your long-term goal. For your first week, these steps might include:

    a. Eat five small meals a day, each containing some healthy fats, complex carbs, and quality proteins.
    b. Complete a cardio workout three days this week, each one consisting of a 30-minute cycling workout covering about 10 miles.
    c. Perform three full-body resistance-training workouts this week.

These behaviors are planned out with a short-term goal in mind: Lose two pounds in the first week (November 1-7). This is a step in the right direction toward achieving your long-term goal of losing 10 pounds by January 1.

Jot down your ideas for the steps in the form of brainstorming notes for now. Don't try to set anything in stone at this stage. You might want to show your ideas to a health and fitness expert who has a good understanding of how feasible and appropriate they are. The next Strategy will help you to narrow down and organize the steps that will form the master plan for your long-term goal.

Strategy 6: Developing a plan of action

How to organize your goals into daily, short-term, and long-term

This Strategy starts off with a scenario for you to visualize:

> The car is packed and you're ready to go on a cross-country trip. From the White Mountains of New Hampshire to the rolling hills of San Francisco, you're excited to see it all. You put the car in gear and off you go. First stop: The Baseball Hall of Fame in Cooperstown, New York. A little while into the trip you need to check the map because you've reached an intersection you're not familiar with. You panic for a moment because you realize you've forgotten your map. But you say the heck with it because you know where you're going. You take a right, change the radio station and keep on going. Unfortunately, you never reach your destination. You waste so much time driving around with no real direction that you miss out on all the great sights you had hoped to see.

Too many of us treat goal-setting the same way: We dream about where we want to go, but we don't have a map to get us there. Do you know what separates having a map from just having a vague idea of the directions? It is the definitiveness of the printed page, along with the ability to see the process of getting from here to there as a series of steps. With a map, you can see where you are in relation to your destination, and you can also see what it will take for you to get there. You know exactly what you are dealing with, and you know that, to get to your destination, you have to follow *all* the in-between steps. Some routes may be quicker than others, but you *have* to pick one and follow it the entire way in order to get where you want to go.

The difference between a dream and a goal parallels the difference between just wanting to go somewhere versus actually having a map so you can see how to do it. A dream focuses on the end result, but when you define it as a goal you are holding yourself accountable to the fact that you have a serious want to achieve it. When you have a goal, you can plan out the steps that you will need to execute in order to reach your desired end. But you need to do more then simply scribble some ideas on a piece of paper. Your goals need to flow from one to another and eventually lead to your desired result, much like a road map. You need to know that, if you follow road A, then road B, and finally road C, you will get where you want to go. This confidence that your goals are waiting at the end of a series of definitive steps will provide you with the motivation to continue on.

Developing a plan of action assignment

1. Look over your notes from the last assignment to see which brainstorming ideas can serve as specific, achievable steps toward a short-term or long-term goal. For example, if your long-term goal will take about a year to reach, you need to have checkpoints (short-term goals) set up at least on a monthly basis. This gives you a goal to shoot for in the not-to-distant future. "Seeing" the end of your short-term goal on the horizon will inspire and energize you. Achieving each goal will infuse you with a sense of accomplishment. In the worst-case scenario, if you miss a short-term target you will have the opportunity to troubleshoot the problem before you fall too far from the path to your long-term goal.

2. Open to the next fresh page in your notebook. Break down your long-term goal into short-term goals that should take no longer than one month for you to reach. You might get ideas from your brainstorming notes from the last Strategy's assignment. List them in the order they will need to be completed, always keeping your long-term goal in the back of your mind. Then break down each of those short-term goals into even shorter periods of time, such as weeks within each month. What needs to be done on a weekly basis?

That's all you need to do at the outset for this assignment. As each week actually approaches you can take a look at the upcoming week and decide what needs to be done on a daily basis. You might get ideas from the brainstorming of specific, achievable steps that you made as part of this assignment. Your best chance for success comes when you have broken the tasks down to the point that you have daily check-ins. There may even be a number of things you need to do each day, depending how high or how numerous your goals are.

Every week you will want to sit down with your notebook and plot out what you need to do for the next seven days. Each night, make sure that you know exactly what you need to do the following day so that nothing's left to chance. These "to-dos" or appointments should go into your day planner to make sure they get done.

To maintain your motivation on a daily basis, you need to understand how each day fits into the big picture. You need to be aware that, if you blow off a day, you will be off-track for achieving your goal in the time frame you had wanted. It is crucial for you to know exactly *what* you have to do, and also to understand the *consequence* of not doing it. The consequence is risking the achievement of your goal, or at least risking the time frame during which you had wanted to achieve it. This is where those pages in your notebook I asked you to paperclip together titled, "How I used to be" might come in handy. Only when you are fully cognizant of the rewards and punishments that may result from your behavior will you truly dedicate yourself to your plan. Having daily accountability to work on your goals will help you stay on track. If personal accountability isn't enough, seek additional support from a family member, friend, mentor, fitness trainer, or personal coach.

Strategy 7: Fine-toothed comb

How to be sure of success

Once you have a draft of your long-term plan, you're going to need to give it some consideration. Make sure there aren't any short-term goals that appear to be too difficult. If there are, you'll want to modify them until everything looks manageable – you'll get a chance to do that in the first assignment for this Strategy. You're much better off being on the conservative side with each short-term goal you make. It's preferable to add more short-term goals if necessary rather than try to make any one short-term goal more difficult. It's fine if each short-term goal is moderately difficult, but none of them should pose a threat to your success. For instance, if you originally set the short-term goal of giving up bread, pasta, and sweets during your first week, but upon thinking it over realize it will be very difficult for you to give all up all three at once, try modifying your short-term goal. You might decide to change your goal to giving up just one of the three items the first week. You can always tackle the other two during another week, but it's ultra-important that you avoid becoming overwhelmed and give up because your goals seem too hard to achieve.

In some cases it might be no problem for you to juggle a handful of short-term goals during the same week, while at other times you might need to focus your attention on one particular goal.

Whether you're focusing on one short-term goal or juggling five, you're usually better off in the long run if all your efforts are geared toward one long-term goal at a time. This means, at any given time, all the short-term goals you're working on should be part of the same long-term goal. You'll find it much harder to manage a bunch of short-term goals when they are part of different long-term goals. It's tougher to maintain your motivation to keep working when your energy is diffused in different directions. You'll see faster progress when you're working toward one master goal. This boosts motivation and makes it less likely that you'll get discouraged.

Furthermore, you'll see faster progress toward your long-term goal if you don't have anything else competing for your attention. The worst thing you can do is allow yourself to become overwhelmed and give up on a goal (unless, of course, you have come to the realization that it's not what you really wanted after all). If you fail to achieve a goal that's important to you, at best you experience a setback, and at worst you stop trying for good. On the other hand, successes build naturally on themselves. Once you develop the confidence that you can attain whatever you set out to do, you will always have the option of setting your sights on larger and larger aspirations if you desire. The opposite holds true as well –

your confidence can spiral downward fast when you experience a setback. That's why it's best to build yourself up by, if anything, keeping your goals on the easy side. You can always "up the ante" on yourself in the future if you like. That isn't always going to be necessary – you should still have fabulous results just being consistent using the slow and steady approach. Let your personal style and preferences dictate how aggressive to be. You *will* reach your final goal eventually as long as you maintain your focus. The only threat to your success lies in losing focus, which can happen quickly if you fail to meet a goal. Therefore, you want to do whatever you can to prevent yourself from losing your momentum.

Now, I realize that most of the time you will have many things going on in your life, and by no means do I want to encourage you to drop everything else in order to focus on one particular long-term goal. However, things will run more smoothly if you allow other areas of your life to stay more or less at status quo while you make a major push in a particular area. It's important to avoid being pulled in too many directions at once. You'll find that you become more efficient in making a change if you hone in on one thing at a time. When you tackle your goals that way, it frees up quite a bit of energy that you can apply to the area you're targeting for change. And when you become more efficient in making a change, you will be able to shift your focus to *another* area that much sooner. Focusing on one thing at a time is really the most efficient way to change your life all-around. Multitasking isn't your best bet in this instance.

Focusing on one thing at a time allows you to remove as many barriers as possible that have the potential to prevent you from achieving your goal. If your goal doesn't require much time and energy because you're using a slow and steady approach, you might find that it's no problem to juggle a handful of goals at once. If you find this to be the case, go for it. Just be sure to add things to your plate one at a time, because that way you'll be able to nip any problems in the bud before you overextend yourself.

Fine-toothed comb assignment

1. Now that you've had time to study this Strategy, go back to the first draft of your plan for your long-term goal and make any necessary changes. You'll be able to look at your draft with a fresh perspective if you take at least 24 hours between completing the draft and looking it over again. Repeat the revising process occasionally as you actually work through your steps. As you try them you will get a better idea of how realistic your original plan was. In hindsight, you might realize that certain steps are a bit too aggressive or a little too easy. You can change your plan as often as needed if things aren't going the way you want. No one gets it right the first time, but if you are persistent and open to change and suggestions you will succeed.

2. It is important that you periodically monitor progress toward your long-term goal. For instance, if your long-term goal is to achieve a "healthy" bodyfat percentage (about 18-25% for females and 15-20% for males), have your bodyfat percentage taken every month. Don't bother having it tested more frequently than that, because it's very hard to detect a significant change in a shorter time frame. Although you can lose up to 1% bodyfat every couple of weeks if you're following a good program, most of the tests carry a margin of error greater than that. Local fitness trainers, athletic trainers, health clinics, and general physicians might offer bodyfat testing.

There are a number of different methods for measuring bodyfat. Don't worry too much about the particular method you use, but understand that you will only be able to detect trends accurately if you stick to the same method from month to month. You also should try to have the same person take your measurement each time for consistency's sake. That way you'll be more likely to detect trends, even if the absolute number is a bit off. You are looking for a ballpark range of accuracy (+/- 4% is the most accuracy that can be hoped for without spending hundreds or thousands of dollars to be tested with sophisticated hospital equipment).

Electronic bodyfat-measuring scales and handheld bodyfat-measuring devices are actually less accurate on average than simple bodyfat calipers. However, as long as you use the same machine each time, the scales and handheld devices should be able to detect trends up or down as long as you take the measurement at the same time of day and in the same physical state. More or less food in your system, dehydration, water retention, and time of day are all confounding factors that can throw off your reading significantly. Skinfold measurements taken with bodyfat calipers are the most accurate test that can be done easily and inexpensively, assuming that you use an experienced tester. You'll get the most accurate readings if you stick with the same tester, same measurement sites, and same skinfold measurement calculation formula from month to month. Another way to track progress is to take girth measurements of your waist, hip, thigh, and any other area that you're interested in changing.

If you have been faithful about working out and eating well but don't see much change in your measurements, keep yourself motivated by noting any progress with your workouts in your exercise log. If you're lifting more weight or running faster this month than you were last month, changes in bodyfat levels are bound to come soon. It may have happened already – there are many factors that can throw your measurements off. A high-sodium meal, use of creatine, and PMS are all instances where you might have enough water retention that you won't be able to detect a drop in bodyfat percentage. If you don't show any changes one month and you know you've been following your program, you'll probably see a double-loss next month (since any loss that happened this month might have been concealed by water retention or some other factor). However, keep in mind that a lack of results, especially over two months' time, might mean that your exercise program and diet need some tweaking, especially if you've been following the same regimen for six weeks or longer.

Don't neglect some type of check-in every month, though, because the information can only help – the truth about what's been happening will either motivate you to continue, or else it will alert you that something is wrong. If you're not getting the results you want, you'll have to face the fact that either you aren't following your program, or else you're going to need to make some changes to it in order to achieve the results you're after.

IV. Taking the Plunge

Now that you've worked your way through the first seven Strategies, you're prepared to start implementing your health and fitness plan. You may have already started thinking about where to work out, how to work out and with whom, and how you will approach your nutrition. Specific advice on these topics is available in this section of the System. You will also find the Reference section in the back of the book helpful as you design your program.

Strategy 8: What's Up Doc?

Consulting with your Physician

If you are generally healthy and see your doctor for a yearly physical, you probably don't need to consult with him specifically to be cleared to start following an exercise and nutrition plan. Odds are your doctor will say, "Go right ahead – that's wonderful, it's just what you need!" Be aware that you will be required to sign a waiver in order to use a gym's facilities or a trainer's services, whether you have been cleared by a doctor or not. Of course, it will never hurt as an added precaution to consult with a physician before starting an exercise program. Most fitness trainers will give new clients a health and fitness evaluation and will alert you if there's something in your evaluation that clearly warrants seeing a physician before starting a new training routine.

If you haven't been active for years, are over age 50, or have a family history of heart problems, it's a different story. In these cases, it's highly recommended that you see your doctor for a check-up and to explain what type of program you are considering. In fact, many health clubs and trainers will require that you do so before you start working out.

And, if you have health problems or take medications you definitely need to check with your doctor before you start an exercise and nutrition program.

What's Up Doc? assignment

1. Decide if you should visit a doctor before you start a new exercise and nutrition plan, and, if so, schedule the appointment as soon as possible.

2. Find out as much as you can about your family's medical history. If you consult with a trainer he will want to know this information. It's also a good idea for you to know your family's medical history so you can choose your goals, workouts, and diet accordingly.

For instance, if your family has a history of heart disease you will definitely want to include cardiovascular exercise in your program and you'll want to follow a diet that's low in saturated fat. If you have a family history of osteoporosis you'll need to pay extra attention to getting enough calcium and you'll need to make resistance training a priority. And, if you have a family history of obesity, and/or diabetes, it should provide further incentive for you to stick with an exercise and diet plan.

Looking through family photo albums can help you pinpoint your genetic body type and give you some clues as to how you might look as you get older (also note the differences between the ones who work out and the ones who don't). All of this information will be useful for setting up your ideal exercise and nutrition plan. You will find specific recommendations in Reference D, "Body Types and Training Recommendations."

Strategy 9: It's a Breeze

How to easily implement your action plan

The most straightforward method for goal implementation is to enter your workouts and food shopping/preparation as appointments or to-dos in your day planner. For some people this provides enough impetus to get everything done. Others do better when they are also held accountable to someone else. If you believe this might be the case for you, have a friend, personal trainer, or other coach check your progress on a daily, or at least weekly, basis.

Rewards are a motivator that can help push you to perform the action steps that are critical for achieving your goals. You should set up your own reward system that is contingent upon specific criteria. For example, you can assign a point value to the behaviors that result in progress toward your goals. For instance, if your goal is weight loss, you might assign a point value to performing your cardio workouts, completing your resistance-training sessions, eating your healthy meals, and taking your supplements. Then you'll need to decide how many points you'll have to accumulate in order to "earn" each reward.

You might decide to have another person give you the reward once you've earned enough points. Or, you can simply reward yourself when the time comes. Some of my personal training clients reward themselves with a facial or a ticket to a ballgame after they've earned a certain number of points. They put a few dollars (one "point" can equal one dollar) in a jar each time they do a workout, for example, and when they've accumulated enough money they go ahead and treat themselves. Your reward will be more powerful if it's something you wouldn't normally have treated yourself to. It will also be more powerful if it's something that is highly motivating for you – your reward should be something that you really, really enjoy.

You definitely want to log your earned points on a *daily* basis and make note of how they are accumulating toward your reward. If you don't award yourself the points you've earned on a *daily* basis, you will miss out on receiving the *immediate* reinforcement that is so critical in maintaining a desired behavior. The points help bridge the gap between the short-term behavior that may feel uncomfortable at times and the long-term benefit that will feel so wonderful once you realize it. The long-term reward of a great body and better health isn't going to come right away, but your points can be awarded on the spot, and you'll know what those points represent – they represent that you've gotten closer to your long-term goal. Human beings are unique "animals" in that we have the capacity to decide to do something for its long-term benefit – we aren't just acting on instinct and impulse. Still, we all are wired to seek pleasure and avoid pain, so you will be better served if you incorporate some type of instant reward into your day to reinforce all the good steps that you're taking. Workout cards or an exercise journal are good ways to keep track of your workout points.

You'll need to put some thought into deciding on the number of points that a certain workout is worth. Taking your personal goals into consideration, the more a specific workout contributes toward your overall progress, the more points that workout should be worth. If you're not sure how different workouts compare, turn to Reference D where you'll see how much weight should be given to specific workouts depending on your body type.

You can also use points to provide extra motivation where it's needed. For instance, if you know that you tend to avoid a certain type of workout even though it would be good for you, bump up the point value of that workout to give yourself more incentive to do it. For instance, if you know that you get a better workout jogging but you always seem to choose the exercise bike over the treadmill, decide to award a 30-minute jog with 4 points and a 30-minute cycling session with just 2. That means you'd have to cycle for twice as long to get the same point value as the jog. Using that point system, do you see why you might be more inclined to choose the jog?

You can use any "token" to keep track of your points. I mentioned that some people use dollar bills, but it really doesn't matter what you use to keep track of your points. However, using tangible objects or "tokens" tends to be more motivating than just seeing numbers or tally marks on paper (tokens are more tangible). A visual display like tokens accumulating in a jar is a tangible way for you to measure progress. Any small object such as a marble or penny works well as a token. If your goal includes a nutrition component, a handy way to track things while you're on the run is to keep a pocketsize notebook with you to log points. Another quick and easy tracking method is to have small index cards with your workouts and your nutrition plan listed on them. You can simply check off your cardio and resistance training workouts as they're completed, and your meals and snacks once you've had them.

I can help you set up a points-based system that includes a training program, a nutrition program, a point-tracking method, appropriate point values for the desired behaviors, and appropriate rewards for your points. All this is included in my complete behavior modification program called Lean Rewards. Your program will be created and completely individualized during a one-on-one consultation. Using expert advice and a proven system like Lean Rewards ensures that your point system will be weighted correctly, meaning that you'll get the fastest results possible given the time and effort you're willing to put into the process. Use my contact information in the back of this book or visit my website www.homeexercisecoach.com if you'd like to learn more about this service.

It's a Breeze assignment

1. Create your own points system, or have one designed for you during a consultation with a qualified trainer or a behavior modification psychologist. Be sure to keep a copy in your notebook or day-planner. You'll find the tables in Reference D helpful if you choose to design your own program because they show the best amount and type of exercise for the various body types. The activities that are weighted more heavily in the table should be awarded with more points.

Think about what you'd like your required number of points per day to be. While you're considering this decision, keep in mind that your points won't represent all work and no play. As you will see if you look at the tables in Reference D, you need to give yourself points for taking scheduled rest days, since rest days are a critical component of achieving optimal health and fitness. You'll learn more about this concept in Strategy 29. In a nutshell, just know that as long as you've worked out on the days you were supposed to, during the past week, your rest days are just as important as your workout days for your overall progress. Therefore, award yourself with the same number of points for resting on a rest day as you'd earn for working out on a workout day. You can certainly take a leisurely walk on a rest day if you like, but avoid doing a formal workout. Also, keep in mind that, if you follow something like the 80/20 Rule with your nutrition, you won't lose points for eating something that's "off" your diet plan as long as you don't go overboard.

Set a minimum quota for the number of points you want to earn per day. You might prefer to take the slow and steady route and just keep hitting that minimum number. Or, if it's your style, some days go above and beyond the minimum in an effort to accelerate your progress.

2. Decide how you'll keep track of your points. Many of my clients using a points system use the token-in-jar method. Some carry pocketsize notepads and make tally marks. Whichever way you keep track, you can transfer your points into your day-planner every week and reward yourself when the time comes.

The key to making the points system work is having a quick and easy way to log your points during the day. Otherwise, the lag time between when you earn the points and when you award them to yourself will make the system a lot less powerful.

Check periodically to be sure that your point tallies do indeed correlate with progress toward your goal (that is, after all, the whole "point" to this entire process! Your points are supposed to reward behaviors that bring you closer to your goal). For example, if you earn 10 points per day on average (2 for a 30-minute cardio session, 2 for a 30-minute resistance-training workout, 1 for taking your multivitamin, 2 for avoiding sugar and white flour, 1 for eating three servings of vegetables, and 2 for not snacking outside of your four planned meals, for instance) but you aren't losing weight or bodyfat, you'll need to consider the criteria you are using for your points. In this particular case, you might need some refining criteria, such as making points contingent upon keeping portions to a certain size, or having your points correlate with workout intensity and not simply workout time (a harder workout is worth more points, judged by an exertion scale that is meaningful to you).

The beauty of the points system is that you can hold yourself accountable to a minimum standard but, at the same time, maintain the flexibility to push yourself further at times for "extra credit." However, you can always be proud just to hit your minimum for the day, because that means you've done your job. This takes some of the pressure off and you will start feeling empowered to accumulate points rather than feel like it's a struggle to keep up the intense pace. This creates more sustained motivation than if you were to feel bad for not doing more and more all the time. Allowing yourself to feel proud of hitting your minimum is a much more positive and action-promoting approach than berating yourself for not being perfect.

Another benefit to the points system is that each day you'll have a fresh start to earn maximum points. This will help keep you motivated on a day-to-day basis. When each day represents a fresh start, you'll realize that the previous day, even if you didn't get many points, is a done deal and you'll get the opportunity all over again to earn more today. Can you see how this will encourage you to put some junk food or a skipped workout behind you and move on? You won't want to give up and let one mistake turn into several when you can "make up" points by doing a little extra the next day to earn some "bonus" points above your minimum.

Having the attitude "today is all that matters" is the key to your long-term success. If you manage to cultivate this attitude in yourself, you'll find yourself making a valiant attempt on a daily basis, and you'll develop the ability to put slips behind you for good. Another great thing about the points system is that, even if your diet falls apart one day, you can "make up for it" by stepping things up on the workout end to pick up some points (or vice-versa – you can make sure your diet is great if you miss a workout). This prevents you from allowing the day, week, or month to be a total waste just because you slipped. It's much harder to have to dig yourself out from a time when you gave up than it is to brush yourself off after a small slip. So many people sabotage themselves because they can't handle not being perfect. If you consistently award yourself for what you do right, you'll find yourself doing those things more and more.

Having a points system allows you to give yourself credit for your positive behaviors even when, like any human being, you're less than perfect. The points system mirrors the way your body responds as well – a few small transgressions off your diet and exercise plan here and there won't affect your progress very much. It's the cumulative effort over time that will get you to where you want to be. The points system teaches you to leave black-and-white thinking behind, allowing you to focus on what you can do *today* to improve your chances of success.

Strategy 10: I'm Obsessed

How to make your goals a positive obsession

If you've been following the strategies you've learned so far, you should find that it's pretty easy to keep your goals on your mind. All the rehearsal and repetition means that things are becoming automatic for you. Imagine how wonderful it will feel when you have all these positive, motivating thoughts and ideas completely engrained in your mind – that is one aspect of the "positive obsession."

Making your goals a positive obsession can also be a conscious decision on your part. At certain times you allow particular aspects of your life to take priority. Assessing priorities is important for your overall success and happiness in life.

To increase your likelihood of having a well-balanced, successful, and satisfying life, you'll need to periodically focus your time and energy on certain aspects of your life. However, this doesn't mean you should let everything else go just because you're focusing on one particular area. People get into trouble when they let everything else go, but they also get into trouble when they try to do too much. You've got to strike the right balance to truly be successful. Try to simply maintain other areas in your life the way they've been going while you make a big push in one particular area.

When you were a teenager your priority might have been sports, school, or a boyfriend or girlfriend. In your 20s it might have been your studies (or maybe it was beer!) If you went to college, even though you probably didn't have a lot of money at the time, you were there with the hope that attaining a degree would lead to a better future. Later in life, building your career and being with your family might have been the big priorities. With so many other things going on, some people don't focus on their health and fitness until it's too late to salvage everything because they've already done irreversible harm to their bodies. Others have always been on top of their fitness in spite of whatever else was going on in their life. Whoever you are and however long you've neglected your body, there's always room for improvement, and you will always benefit by making exercise and eating healthy a part of your life.

There is never a time when you can justify not doing at least the minimum with exercise and eating right. There are simply too many benefits to pass up. Luckily, diet and exercise don't have to be all encompassing – you can certainly keep them near the top of your priority list while maintaining a full life that includes work, family, friends, spirituality, and plenty of fun. Taking the time to improve your health and fitness will actually improve your life all around. You'll feel better, be more productive, and enjoy a ton of stress relief. In the end you will have *more* time to do what you want, and you'll have more *quality* years due to improved health and vitality if you take the time to exercise and eat well. In other words, you'll not only live longer, but you'll also be healthier and more active during those years. That being said, I'll be the first to admit that getting into the swing of things can be tough – indeed, the hardest part of any health and fitness program is getting started.

Take a look at where your priorities lie right now, and make the decision to give health and fitness a relatively high rank in your life. The order in which you rank your priorities will depend on your particular circumstances. Decide just how important improving your health, fitness, and appearance is to you right now, and also figure out how important that is in relation to other things in your life. Once you do this you'll know what, if anything, needs to get "bumped" in order to accommodate the time it will take to get and stay healthy and fit.

If exercise and eating right are high on your priority list, you'll schedule those things into your life first, not last. Figure out when your energy level tends to be highest during the day, and schedule your workouts at that time whenever possible.

Convenience is a huge issue when it comes to working out and eating right. If you are able to stop at a gym that's on the way home rather than have to drive in the other direction, you will have a much easier time sticking to your plan. If you are extremely busy (and who isn't these days?) you might find that working out at home is the best option. It's not for everyone, but I've seen countless people get into phenomenal shape exercising at home, even if they have access to little or no equipment. It's nice to have a full gym because you'll have more options, but a home gym costing thousands is certainly not necessary to get in great shape. If you decide to work out at home, you can invest in a few inexpensive pieces of equipment for your "gym" every year, and before you know it you'll have a nice little setup for yourself.

An adequate home gym doesn't have to cost more than a few hundred dollars even for an advanced exerciser, assuming that you'll be able to do cardiovascular work outside. Even if you'll need to do your cardio indoors, you can use an inexpensive aerobic step for your cardio, or you can do your resistance training in a circuit format, which can take the place of cardio because it gets your heart rate up and burns a good number of calories. An exercise bike or a bike stand for your outdoor bike (so you can use it indoors) are also fairly inexpensive cardio options. If money isn't an issue, consider purchasing an elliptical trainer or a treadmill so you'll have the option to do indoor cardio. You'll need to spend at least $500, but probably $1,000 or more to get a good-quality treadmill or elliptical trainer. A lower-cost option is a portable lateral stepper that can be purchased at many sporting goods stores for about $125.

To make eating well a snap, plan for food shopping and meal-preparation during a low-key time in your week. That way you'll be sure to have supplies on hand, as well as some meals and snacks already prepared for times when you need something in a pinch. Lack of time and lack of planning are the top two reasons why people abandon healthy eating. Assuming you have a smartly designed diet plan that doesn't cut calories too low, the only other reason you'd give healthy eating is because your good behavior isn't being rewarded immediately (the change in appearance and increased sense of well-being generally take place over time, not right away). When you eat "right" but miss eating all the things you used to, in the short-term you experience pain with no apparent reward, which isn't helpful at all for reinforcing desired behavior. The points system I described in the last Strategy should help you overcome this problem by providing instant gratification when you do the right things.

Your life will become ten times easier once you have systems in place to direct it. By this point, hopefully you've done the assignments and developed your own version of the systems I've explained in the Strategies. After you've taken the time to design your program using the guidelines in this book, following through with everything is the easy part. All you will need to do at that point is follow the instructions you've created for yourself. Eventually you might not need to track your points or follow the systems so religiously because doing the right things will have become second nature. Until that time comes, you'll need to be conscious and particular about what you're doing at all times in order to keep yourself on track. If you don't want to go through all the bother, you might consider working closely with a trainer who can design everything for you. I have some clients who choose to do this and they are pretty happy with the arrangement. If you want to take control of as much as possible on your own, that's certainly a fine approach too, and one that will save you some money on training. Even though working with a trainer a few times a week usually means quicker results for you, it's certainly not a requirement for seeing great results, and a motivated person working on his own usually does better than an unmotivated one working with a trainer.

The bottom line is that you will need to take some responsibility for pushing yourself, whether you are working with a trainer regularly or not.

Through offering a System like this, I hope that some of you will feel empowered to take control of many aspects of your health and fitness, leaving me in the position to act mainly as a consultant and program designer. Now don't get me wrong – I love having clients I see multiple times per week for continuous training, but I know that's not realistic financially for everyone, or even desired by everyone. Some people enjoy having their workout time to themselves and prefer to train alone most of the time.

As far as I'm concerned, there are four principal components to the job of a personal fitness trainer:

1. Education on how to get fit
   –for clients and the public at large
2. Program Design
   – the exercise routine and proper nutrition
3. Motivation
   –serving as a motivator and also helping you find your own sources of motivation
4. Personal Service
   –customer service surpassing expectations, cultivating trust, and developing strong relationships

Personally, I have begun to pay special attention to the education and program design facets of my business as it grows, since those are the areas where I feel that I offer the most value to all potential clients. It's also the area where I can best leverage my time since I can only see so many clients in a given day, but I can reach many more through programming and educational materials. Of course, I understand the need to use trainers for motivation and personal service as well, which is why one of my business goals is to employ trainers who will provide the bulk of our continuous training services to clients. By teaching my methodology to other trainers and stepping up advertising and publicity to attract more clients, I will be able to reach more people with my message and my philosophy. I'm sure to pick up some good tips and ideas from my staff as well. My overriding business goal is to be constantly improving the perceived value of the products and services my business offers.

Although education and program design are going to be my primary focus as a trainer and business owner, motivation and personal service/relationships are definitely key as well, and for many clients can mean the difference between sticking with a program and dropping out. Why else, with all the diet and exercise advice out there, do so many people still struggle with their health and fitness? While education and program design help bring in new clients, motivation and personal service/relationships keep clients coming back, assuming of course that they're getting results from their program. That's why I know my business has to be strong on each of the four components if I want to continue having a thriving business and happy clients.

I'm Obsessed assignment

1. Reference A, "The 10 Tricks You Need to Know to Eat Right, one person at a time" provides an example of how to set up a system for success. That article happens to discuss systems for your nutrition. Read through Reference A and follow the tips that you think might be helpful to you. If you follow these guidelines, you will find it much easier to have healthy food prepared and on hand, even if you are preparing food just for one. If you live alone or prepare two sets of meals, these tips for making the preparation of diet-friendly foods quick and easy will really come in handy. When you have everything you need on hand when you need it, you'll be able to easily and conveniently make the dietary choices that will help you achieve your goals. You'll also be able to take responsibility for your own diet by not leaving yourself susceptible to being influenced by forces in your environment. If you know how to cook healthy for one, you'll never be able to fall back on the excuse that you couldn't eat well because your family was eating something fattening or because everyone decided to order out.

2. Having a social support system can make all the difference in your success, especially during the first weeks of a program. Find a friend, family member, or trainer who you can lean on for support, at least during your initial 30-day commitment. By that point, hopefully you will have established your "positive obsession" and you will find it much easier to stay with your program. However, if you are a socially oriented person you will probably find that you always do better when you have ongoing support from others. Call for more information on my popular "Jump Start Your Fitness" program if you'd like my help in getting off on the right track.

   An extremely powerful tactic for keeping yourself on track is to tell others about your program and your goals. This is a highly effective technique for a number of reasons. Explaining your program to others helps you reinforce in your own mind what you are doing and why. When you become a "teacher" you tend to become a better student. Once you have explained your program and the rationale behind it to others, you will understand it better yourself. You will also start to feel social pressure to appear to be consistent in front of other people. To appear to be consistent, you must actually do what you say you will do. Your pride will be at stake to "practice what you preach." If you don't, others might start to look down on you for it. In other words, you start feeling accountable to follow through when others know your intentions.

3. You can also help foster the "obsession" by reading books, magazines, and articles about fitness and nutrition. This will help keep your mind "on topic." Recommended sources are listed in Reference E, and the links can be found on my website, www.homeexercisecoach.com.

Strategy 11: A spoonful of sugar

How to create a supportive exercise atmosphere

You will be happiest and most successful if your workouts and diet are convenient and enjoyable. You'll need to decide where you'd like to work out, what type of workout you'd like to do, the best social atmosphere for you, and the frequency of workouts you'd like to shoot for. You should choose your workout schedule based on a combination of what is most efficient and what is most effective, and also on any special needs or considerations you may have.

No exercise, no matter how good, is worth doing if you hate it or if it aggravates an injury. Unless you are looking to get in model-caliber shape or compete in high-level athletics, you shouldn't have to do any type of exercise that you absolutely despise. Investigate your options and allow yourself a trial period to see if something works for you. A fitness trainer can help you make these decisions because the trainer will be familiar with a wide range of training modalities and probably has experience working with someone who comes from a similar background. A good trainer can usually detect before the fact when something might lead to injury, and can offer alternatives for an exercise if something isn't working well for you. The bottom line, however, is that there will always be trial and error involved as you settle on what keeps you happy and also results in steady progress.

A spoonful of sugar assignment

1.   Shop around for health clubs, gyms, or personal training studios where you might want to work out. Try working out at home and see how you like it. Experiment with taking your cardiovascular exercise outdoors, using cardio machines at the gym or at home, and trying some group classes. Decide what will make you happiest and give you the best workout, whether that means sticking to one option for a while or using a combination of things to get your exercise. Decide if you'd like to work with a trainer and, if so, how frequently. Finally, decide if you'd like to train with a workout partner for some or all of your workouts.

2.   Buy yourself some nice workout gear so you feel good while you work out. If your budget is tight, the most important purchase is good-quality footwear specifically designed for the activity you plan to do. For instance, if you walk for exercise you shouldn't wear running sneakers – if you do, you'll be asking for trouble with your feet. Shoes that are designed with a particular activity in mind are constructed to offer the most support during a specific motion – such a jumping, walking, or lateral motion. I'm not a big fan of "cross-trainers" because they aren't the ideal shoe for any particular activity. If you really need to perform more than one activity wearing the same shoes, skip the "cross-trainers." Instead, go for the most basic running shoe you can find. A basic running shoe won't have fancy features that could prove to be problematic for other activities.

Also, realize that the footwear you've worn during exercise for the past 3-6 months generally won't provide much support and should be replaced, unless you are one of the lucky few that could even exercise barefoot with no problems. If this is the case, you probably didn't need the support of the shoes anyway, and could probably get away with wearing them for longer than the recommended 3-6 months.

If you have special foot issues such as high arches or excessive pronation or supination (feet rolling in or out, respectively), you should use shoes specifically designed to correct for those problems. A specialty shoe store such as a runner's outlet should have staff on duty that can help you find the right shoes. You also might try looking at the websites of some of the major shoe brands such as Asics, New Balance, and Saucony. Those websites have resources to help you figure out which foot type you have, and allow you to perform a search to find the shoe models that are appropriate for your foot type. Armed with this information, you'll be able to go into any store and have some idea of what you need. This comes in handy when there isn't any knowledgeable staff member on duty, a situation you'll tend to encounter in large chain stores.

If you've been wearing the right type of shoe and still experience problems, you might have a more serious foot issue that requires custom orthotics to correct. Keep this in mind if you continue to experience foot or leg pain while exercising. Although foot and leg pain are the most common problems when you wear sneakers that don't suit your needs, all areas of the body, especially the low back, can be affected. Make sure you're working out with the right footgear, because it can make all the difference in your comfort and safety during a workout.

3. After the decisions about workout type, workout location, and workout gear have been made, the next thing you need to do is create a supportive exercise atmosphere by surrounding yourself with people who encourage you. Furthermore, try to surround yourself with others who follow a healthy lifestyle themselves. Ask your friends and family who don't work out or who have been working out by themselves to join you one day. Try going on an "exercise date" with your significant other, whether this involves going to the gym together, going for a bike ride, playing tennis, or hiking. You'll probably find that your bond with other people grows stronger when you exercise together. Get together with a friend or two to go for a walk so you can catch up with each other and get some exercise at the same time.

If there are people in your life who don't support your new lifestyle changes and talking to them doesn't work, try to associate with them as little as possible. You don't want to let their negative energy drag you down.

Strategy 12: Decisions, decisions

Choosing your health and fitness resources

There are many books and magazines available to help you learn more about health and fitness. Be choosy with what you read, however, because not all of them are based on sound, scientifically proven advice. Avoid materials that focus on a fad or gimmick. Also, if the article makes outrageous claims, it's a tip-off that the advice is questionable. Basically, when something seems too good to be true, it probably is.

Also, keep in mind that many exercise and nutrition books, magazines, and websites serve are thinly disguised advertisements for particular brands of supplements. You will be able to pick out these articles because they are written with the purpose of building up a health or fitness problem, and, according to the article, a particular brand's supplement happens to be the ideal solution. That's not to say that the information isn't valid – it may or not be accurate. However, a company with supplement sales at stake is likely to embellish claims, use misleading statistics, or report statistics from a biased study that might be funded by their own company. These articles and ads will tell you that the best (or only) solution to the particular health and fitness issue in question is to purchase their supplement. Consider it a red flag if the article fails to give you a complete picture of all your options. And if it blasts some of the "solutions" while really talking up one in particular, you can be willing to bet that their publication is little more than a sales pitch.

That being said, I recommend the following books as relatively bias-and-agenda-free sources of fitness information:

–Beyond Brawn by Stuart McRobert
–BodyBuilding 101: Everything You Need to Know to Get the Body You Want by Robert Wolff, Ph.D

These books have exercises and workout routines that can be used as part of a muscle-building or fat-loss program.

In the periodical department, I recommend the following:

–Robert Kennedy's Oxygen Women's Fitness
–Men's Fitness and Health
–Home Bodies Monthly
(had to throw in that plug…)

I must give a general warning on fitness magazines: If you're looking for straightforward information, you'll probably find the magazines to be more confusing than helpful. In order for all the health and fitness magazines to produce a new issue each month, they need to come up with lots of variations on a handful of common themes. That's the only way they'll be able to keep the material fresh. They also need to differentiate themselves somehow – if every magazine printed only the best material month after month, there wouldn't be any incentive to buy one title over the other. A magazine geared toward your particular demographic (women in their 30s and 40s, men wanting to bulk up, etc.) will lead you to believe it's stuff is the latest and greatest and is specified to suit your needs. The fact of the matter is that "basics" are called basics for a reason – you can add to them, but you can't skip them and you're never "beyond" them. You simply can't get around following their principles unless you have enviable genetics that allow you to look great even if you *don't* exercise in the most effective manner.

See, the sad fact is that many of the variations you see between physiques have more to do with genetics than anything else. Also, diet, supplements, and drugs are at least as important as training protocol in terms of the way your body looks, assuming of course you're performing a general resistance-training program with sufficient frequency and intensity. The main difference between the recommendations for a person looking to gain muscle and a person looking to lose fat is that the "gainer" will need to increase his calorie intake and the "loser" will need to reduce his. They both need to weight-train, usually in the 6-12-rep range, and they both need a good amount of protein in their diet – if anything, the dieter needs *more* weight training and a *higher* protein intake as a percentage of his diet than someone looking to build mass (assuming the lifter is "natural," i.e. not on steroids or andro). Looking through the magazines, it is tough to decipher such simple truths amongst all the hype.

I understand what the editors are doing, because I realize that if the magazines got to the point and gave you the fundamentals you needed to know, they would put themselves right out of business. Most of the information in these magazines is accurate in some sense – the material just tends to have a slant to it or a new spin put on it that's not really necessary or is easily misinterpreted. Quite often the articles fail to tell both sides of a story in a straightforward manner, which is important if a reader wants be educated and not simply entertained. That's what I try to do with my Newsletter – *hopefully* it's entertaining to read, but my priority is to educate you on health and fitness issues and make sure that you understand both sides of a story. Certainly some readers *are* simply looking to be entertained, which is why there's a place for those types of magazines. Since you are this far into the book, it's probably safe for me to assume that *your* main priority in reading health and fitness materials is to be educated and to change your body for the better.

You can use the health and fitness magazines for workout and nutrition ideas, but try not to get hung up on the "latest thing" and let your focus shift too far away from the fundamentals of exercise and nutrition. Fad workouts and diets will come and go, but dumbbells, barbells, and a nutritious diet have been around forever, and people will continue going back to them no matter what new innovation comes out. The books and magazines that I've recommended in this Strategy are better than most I've seen at getting to the truth and leaving out unnecessary fluff and meaningless hype.

There are some excellent websites that can help you design routines and increase your fitness and nutrition knowledge. For your convenience, these links can be found on my website, http://www.homeexercisecoach.com. In case you'd like to go to them directly, here are a few websites that I recommend:

–http://www.stumptuous.com/weights.html
This one is written for women, but it's the best beginner fitness and nutrition site that I've seen, and the advice is applicable to both genders.

–http://www.fitnessonline.com
Good for general health and fitness info.

–http://www.intense-workout.com/map.html
Good for diet and exercise plans specifically designed to help you build muscle and/or lose fat.

www.bodyrecomposition.com
This site is for the advanced exerciser who doesn't mind a technical/science bent (it's still written in everyday language) and is interested in the theory of training and nutrition, cyclic dieting, and the integration of training and nutrition. I use this site all the time to get ideas for my own diet and workouts. The author Lyle McDonald is as knowledgeable as they come.

In addition, I hope you will consider me to be your ultimate resource for all the fitness information you could ever need. My phone and email are always open to my readers, customers, and clients. All the links I've recommended can be found on my website, www.homeexercisecoach.com. I will be adding links and valuable content to my site as often as I can, making it a great fitness resource for you with all the content fully screened and endorsed by me. You can also subscribe to my newsletter, purchase a select assortment of supplements I recommend, and purchase additional copies of this book on the website.

If you decide to hire a fitness trainer, there are several issues to think about. It is preferable that your trainer has a good amount of experience working in the field and can provide testimonials from past and present clients, along with their contact information if you request it. It's always a plus if he is nationally certified and/or has a degree in exercise physiology. Ask if he specializes in specific issues that are important to you (examples of specialties as a trainer include weight management, psychology of training, bodybuilding, functional training, post-rehabilitation, and sport-specific training). Find out if he has worked with other clients who had similar needs to yours, and what their outcomes were.

None of that matters much, however, if you don't like and enjoy working with your trainer. This is something that you'll have to discover for yourself by trying a trainer on for size. Ask if he offers a free consultation or a money-back guarantee to protect your investment if things don't work out.

Not all trainers offer a free consultation, and that is based more on their business philosophy than anything else. Some trainers want to maintain a high fee associated with their time, while others figure that everyone is better off if a client can sample the services before he buys. A trainer's rates do not seem to correlate tremendously with his level of expertise, nor with the typical results his clients get. They *are* related to his business structure, pricing philosophy, target clientele, geographical location, and venue for delivering services. If a trainer works for a gym, he might not have control over the rate he charges. You might find a trainer who offers a lower-cost introductory package to encourage people to sample his services. Regular rates for most trainers working in suburbs out of gyms or studios are typically $50-$65 an hour. In-home appointments and trainers in major metropolitan areas tend to run a bit higher.

If this seems like a lot of money to spend on a regular basis, keep in mind that most trainers offer a choice between continuous training services and consulting services. With continuous training, you meet with the trainer at least once per week. The trainer stays with you through a workout and gives you direction as to what to do for workouts and/or nutrition when you're on your own. On the other hand, if you use a trainer strictly for consulting you might meet as little as twice per year, although as a general rule you'd meet with the trainer once per month. With monthly appointments the trainer can test your bodyfat percentage, address any concerns you may have, and otherwise evaluate progress before too much time has gone by. You'll discuss how the last month went and you can get your form and routine checked. A month is also right around the time when you'd want to make a change to your program to allow for the fastest progress in the upcoming month.

Some trainers offer appointments of various lengths, while others always charge by the hour. Training consultations over the phone and via email are becoming increasingly popular with those who want personalized advice without having to deal with travel time or scheduling conflicts. I offer this service for some of my clients who are comfortable with the form for most exercises and just want some accountability and guidance. I'll still meet with them in person on occasion to take measurements and conduct form checks, but for the most part those clients just use me for consulting and perform most of their workouts on their own.

You'll need to make sure that the trainer you're considering offers a wide selection of days and hours for appointments and has enough room in his schedule to accommodate you. Be aware that, if you opt to use continuous training services, it is common practice for a trainer to request that you commit to a set schedule for the month, if not longer. Most aren't doing this to "rope you in" to a contract – it's just easier for everyone if both parties can make every attempt to stick to a consistent schedule. Having set schedules also allows trainers to see as many clients during their workday as possible. It streamlines billing and enables us to offer you more time slots while helping us keep our rates down. If I can only fit four clients into my workday because everyone keeps changing the training time he wants, I will be tempted to charge more just so I can make a decent living. Personally, I am committed to providing top-notch customer service, so my business offers everything from early morning to late evening as well as some weekend appointments. It makes things a bit more complicated to manage on my end, but I feel that every client should be able to choose an appointment time that works well for him. In order for me to offer that flexibility, however, I need to know in advance when people will train.

One of the latest trends in the industry is the money-back guarantee for personal training services. This demonstrates that the trainer stands behind his advice and expertise, and also serves as insurance for you so that you won't risk throwing your money away on bad advice. This is especially important since, at the time of this printing, the personal fitness training industry is not formally regulated. There are a number of certification and degree programs for personal trainers, but there is still no nationally accepted standard for who can call himself a trainer. This means that one "certified personal trainer" or CPT might have taken an entirely different course and test than another CPT. Industry regulation for personal fitness professionals is a hot topic today and is on the horizon for the near future. A national accreditation standard is slated to be in place by December 31, 2005.

Decisions, decisions assignment

1. Decide whether you want to use books, magazines, the Internet, a trainer, or some combination of these resources for your health and fitness information and as a way to keep abreast with the latest updates. You don't want to waste your time, money, and effort exercising and paying attention to your nutrition unless you are sure that the techniques you're using are effective. Start utilizing various resources to expand your fitness and nutrition knowledge. Reading and using this System is a great start. You can review section II, "The 7 Keys to Raising Your Metabolism for Life," and take a look at the Reference section toward the end of the book for some fundamental training and diet advice.

It is critically important that you have a strong foundation in the basics. Sometimes people complain that the basic exercises are boring. If boredom is a problem, I'll think up a few variations I can give the client to satisfy his need for variety, but I also take the time to explain the rationale behind my routine design.

The first thing you need to understand is that every beginner should perform a full-body resistance-training program 2-3 times per week for best results. That routine should include a basic exercise for each major muscle group. Couple this notion with the fact that certain exercises have proven to be superior to other exercises for targeting a particular muscle group. This brings us to my dilemma – *Unless I am willing to give some of my beginner clients a second-rate exercise, of course they are all going to do virtually the same thing!*

I've seen trainers who are all about "the latest hype" – their clients are playing with all kinds of gizmos and gadgets and doing things that look "neat." That's fine and dandy if your primary goal is to be entertained while you exercise, but most clients come to me wanting to get in the best shape they can. If this is not the primary goal for a particular client, I will find out during the initial consultation and will cater his program accordingly to incorporate more "fun" training into the mix. I have no problem with that if the client is willing to accept substandard results for the sake of having more "fun" while training.

However, I flat-out refuse to give my clients anything but the best in accordance to his goals – I take a client's goals seriously. I adopt his goals as my own when I agree to take him on as a client. Only once a client is a couple of months into the game will more variations be warranted. Ironically, the individuals who get "bored" easily are the ones who don't tend to stick it out long enough to get past the beginner stage. It's ironic because, after the first couple of months, it *does* make sense to incorporate more variety into the training sessions. The problem with using a lot of variety with beginner clients is twofold: there is a learning curve for picking up the correct form on the movements, and also for neurologically conditioning the muscles to a particular movement. Only once these two components are established will you be able to get the most out of an exercise. Furthermore, it doesn't make sense to use lots of variety with a beginner who simply doesn't need it yet to see results, because it's better to "save" the variety for later when you reach a plateau with your original program. If you go through most of the "tricks" right away, you won't have as much opportunity to change things in the future. "If it ain't broke, don't fix it" is a good mantra to follow with your fitness. If a program continues to give you results, there is no need to change anything. However, almost everyone will see their progress stall eventually if they never make a change to their program.

In spite of the fact that it would be "neat" and "exciting" for me too if I gave everyone different stuff, I resist the temptation. I know that sticking with the proven game plan will be worth it on the day my client comes to me absolutely glowing from all the compliments he's been getting.

V. The Daily Grind

Starting your health and fitness plan is half the battle. Now that you've begun to implement you health and fitness plan, you're ready to learn helpful tips and techniques to make your program more effective and help things run smoothly. In this section you'll find specific advice on basic health and fitness topics.

Strategy 13: If you fail to plan, you plan to fail

How to rehearse for success

The title for this Strategy pretty much says it all. I've already talked quite a bit about planning, so there isn't much more I can say on the topic without being redundant. Still, planning is such an important concept that it deserves it's own Strategy.

I'd like to emphasize the main benefit you get from planning, which is that you get to be *proactive* instead of *reactive*. Being proactive means that you decide what you'd like to do and then you act on it. You take full responsibility for the fact that you are the one who dictates the course for your life. When you're in reactive mode you're just responding to what is happening around you. You never feel in control of your life, and you don't get to enjoy the sense of freedom that goes along with doing what *you* want to do. A proactive person takes each day by the horns, while a reactive person lets each day pass him by. If you're reactive, you run from one thing to the next simply acting in response to what's happening around you. It's not a very fulfilling existence, nor one that readily lends itself to happiness and success. This Strategy's assignments cover some additional ground on planning. They will guide you in generating some ideas so that you can enjoy even more of the benefits that come from thorough planning. If you plan what you need to do, you're much more likely to get the results you want.

Still not sure planning is worth it? According to a recent study on women and success, women who consider themselves to be very successful share characteristics and attitudes that contrast sharply with those who don't (6). For example, 76% of women who called themselves "very successful" say they often set personal goals and make specific plans for achieving them, while only 46% of the less successful women said the same. 47% of very successful women say they make lists all the time, versus just 34% of less successful women (And 43% of the very successful women exercise a few times a week, compared to only 26% of the less successful women).

All this hard work and planning seems to pay off. Those who called themselves "very successful" had a median household income of $70,800, while women who said that their level of success was average or below average had a median household income of $53,200.

If you fail to plan, you plan to fail assignment

1. Make sure that you have each day planned out before it begins so that you don't get caught by surprise with no time left to exercise and eat right.

2. If you catch yourself obsessing about something in the past, or about what *could* go wrong, make a conscious effort to turn your thinking around. Keep your mind filled with positive thoughts and visualize things going well.

3. Take a moment to summon your energy and clear your mind before your workouts. Include a warm-up to prepare your mind and body for what's to come. A proper warm-up consists of 5-10 minutes of easy cardio, such as pedaling a bike, walking, or slow stair-stepping. Spend that time letting go of any stress you may be carrying and think about your goals for your workout.

4. Always have the food you'll need to follow your nutrition plan on hand. Stock up when you can, and keep some non-perishables in your desk or in the car. See Reference A, "The 10 Tricks You Need to Know to Eat Right, one person at a time" for more tips on planning as it relates to sticking to a healthy diet.

5. Make sure to leave enough time carved out for your workouts – you don't want to rush yourself. If you're rushed, you'll miss out on the stress reduction following a workout and the sense of well-being and relaxation that you'd normally experience afterward. Moreover, you simply won't perform as well when you feel rushed. When you're rushed, you're less likely to use proper control while lifting weights, and your heart rate will be affected by the anxiety, which means you won't get as much benefit from the exercise.

6. Always have a "Plan B." For example, familiarize yourself with a home exercise routine in case you aren't able to get to the gym one day. Know some alternate exercises for all the major muscle groups if you find yourself having to use different equipment or if you need to rest an injury. Keep nutritious staples at home that you can whip up into a healthy meal in case you run out of fresh ingredients.

Strategy 14: Hocus Focus

How to concentrate during exercise and eating to maximize results

It's extremely important for you to learn and master the mind-to-muscle connection. Having the mind-to-muscle connection means that you're able to isolate the muscles you're trying to work during each exercise. You should be able to pinpoint which muscles are being placed under stress during an exercise, and you should have the ability to direct the focus to the muscles you want to work. If you don't know where you *should* be feeling a certain exercise, consult a trainer or an exercise manual.

You should be able to feel your level of fatigue increase during the set, but at the same time feel in control of the weight and your rep speed. Concentrate on cues that help you maintain the correct form. One or two-word cues tend to work best. For example, "elbows in" works better than, "keep the elbows close by the body." The shorter cue gets right to the point, which means you can make the correction sooner. Not everyone will need the same form tips and cues to do the exercises correctly, so you'll need to learn the aspects of form to which you need to pay special attention. A trainer or an exercise manual can help you hone in on the aspects that tend to give you trouble.

It's also important that you use the appropriate level of exertion during resistance training to get the most benefit. Score yourself on perceived exertion, letting 0 be no exertion and 10 be complete failure of the muscle ("Failure" means that your muscles simply give up at the end of the set). If you're a beginner, stay at level 3-4 on perceived exertion during your first week or two of workouts.

By your third week, try working out at level 5-6. At this level you should feel like you're putting forth a good amount of effort, but still not feel highly fatigued or drained. At level 5-6, you shouldn't lose your breath during the workout, and you should feel like you *could* do more if you tried to.

After you've been working out consistently for about six weeks, try to work out at level 6-7 most of the time. If you're interested in pushing yourself further, try bumping it up to level 8-9 once a week. At that level, you will be on the brink of muscular failure during weight training and your heart rate will be up as high as is tolerable for you to sustain during cardio. Most people find that working out at this level once a week is plenty because it requires so much physical and mental energy. Working out at this level can drain you quite a bit – in fact, you'll probably want to rest the muscle groups you worked at that level for a couple of days. You might not even feel like exercising at all the following day, which is fine because a rest day is the perfect follow-up to a high-intensity workout.

Think twice before you attempt to work out at level 10. For cardio, level 10 might consist of all-out interval sprints as fast as you can go, alternated with short recovery periods at a slower pace. For resistance training, level 10 might involve performing forced reps (reps using another person's assistance *after* the point at which you hit muscular failure during a set). It's necessary to work at this level of intensity once in a while if you're aiming to be in phenomenal shape, but it is *not* necessary to be fit. If you really want to get into great shape, however, you will need to push yourself to that degree at times.

Even if you're trying to be realistic about the level of fitness you can attain, don't rule out high-intensity sessions if you're up for a challenge. When you push yourself you'll get more out of the time you spend exercising. That's the reason I encourage my clients to try forced reps and other intensity techniques once in a while. For safety reasons, never attempt a super-challenging set without a spotter, and avoid performing all-out interval sprints if you're by yourself.

The most reasonable thing to do is to take at least one day of rest from exercise following your intense workouts. That will give your body the necessary time for recovery to ensure that you get all the muscular and metabolic adaptation you can out of your workout. It's the day *after* the workout that your body actually gets stronger, and by avoiding stressful activity for 24 hours after that tough session your body will be able to apply all of its resources toward responding to the training. If you take the time and effort to work out, it's silly to not allow yourself sufficient rest so that you can get the most out of it! Taking a rest day after such an intense effort is also smart because you're more likely to injure yourself during training when you've fatigued yourself to that degree during the past few days. You won't be as strong, fresh, or alert during physical activity for a day or two following such an intense effort.

Hocus Focus assignment

1. It's going to take a bit of work to establish your mind-to-muscle connection. However, once you've got it, you shouldn't have to think much about it anymore.

To start working on your mind-to-muscle connection, the first step is to put all distractions out of your mind while you are working out. Follow the tips in the second paragraph of this Strategy as you work to develop the mind-to-muscle connection for the exercises you plan to do.

Keep in mind that you will perform best on new or difficult tasks if you have no distractions. On the other hand, if you are doing something routine, distractions will have the opposite effect. Distractions will actually improve your performance in that instance because they help fight boredom. Therefore, during your easier, more routine workouts, you can read or use headphones while you exercise once you know you've established the mind-to-muscle connection for the muscles you're targeting.

When you're using intensity techniques like forced reps during resistance training, your mind needs to be completely in tune with your body. This means you should keep distractions to a minimum so you can remain focused on what you're doing.

When it comes to tough cardio workouts, some people will perform best if they have no distractions, while others do better with some distraction because it takes their mind off the effort and makes the time pass faster. Cardio doesn't require the same type of mind-to-muscle connection as weights, and the level of exertion with cardio isn't as high. That's why most people can listen to music or read during intense cardio and still perform very well. In fact, the distraction might help you push harder and longer because intense cardio, although not resulting in muscular failure like the weights, can be uncomfortable and tough to get through at times.

2. Good nutrition also requires concentration. You need to be conscious of the types and quantities of foods you choose and conscious of the effects they will have on your body. You'll find that it pays off to remain mindful while eating. If you pay close attention, your body will tell you what type and how much food it needs. Your body will also tell you when it's had enough. Avoid reading, watching TV or using the computer while you're eating. Sometimes your body will be full but your brain won't realize it's had enough until it's too late and you've already overeaten. The faster you eat

and the more distractions you have while eating, the greater the "lag time" you'll have between the point when you've physically had enough food and point at which your body and brain realize it. This window of "lag time" can be dangerous for your weight because it's the time when you're most likely to overeat.

**Strategy 15: Short-Term Sacrifice –
Food Cravings and Exercise Avoidance**

**How to overcome the need for instant gratification
that will sabotage your success**

Human beings, like all "animals," are wired to seek instant gratification. Our instincts drive us toward going after what we can get in the short term – that is, we tend to choose what will give us the greatest amount of pleasure and the least amount of pain in the immediate future. Sure, we have the *capacity* to do what we know is best for us, even if it doesn't feel very good at the time. That doesn't mean it's easy to make the right choices, though. Only by becoming *obsessed* with achieving our long-term goals will it become painful enough for us to fall short of them that we're willing to bypass the short-term gratification that stands in the way of our success. The pain we feel as a result of failing to achieve our long-term goals can be a strong motivator for us to do what we need to do in the short-term to reach them.

However, it is not enough just to cause ourselves to feel pain if we don't achieve our goals. It is critical to our success that we *make the actual process of achieving them* as pleasurable and reward-laden as possible. Rewarding yourself when you do the right things is one way to accomplish this. Also, the more informed you are about health and fitness the better equipped you will be to make exercise and eating right less painful and more pleasurable. You don't need to have the "no pain, no gain" mentality in order to do well. Sure, there will be times when you will feel uncomfortable while getting in shape, but if you can achieve the same result with less pain, more power to you! The fact that you didn't have to suffer every step of the way doesn't take away from your accomplishment. I admire the person who figures out a way to get the same result with less pain – it's silly to make exercise more painful than it needs to be to get results.

Not sure how to make diet and exercise less painful? With diet, there are certain ways of eating that can help prevent hunger and increase the satisfaction you get from your diet while you're losing weight. To make the exercise component less painful overall, the concept of having "easy" days and "rest" days fits the bill, and you'll learn more about the benefits of easy days and rest days in Strategy 29. There are many effective tactics out there, and you'll find that, for you, some will work better than others. Because everyone responds differently, there are few hard and fast rules.

One tip that seems to be helpful for everyone is to include plenty of high-fiber foods in your diet. A high fiber intake helps keep you feeling full while dieting. Whole grains, legumes, fruits, and vegetables are all good sources of fiber. If you get 2-4 servings of whole grains or lentils and at least 5 servings of fruits and vegetables per day, you should have no problem getting the recommended amount of dietary fiber. Fiber supplements are an option if you struggle to get the recommended 25-30 grams of dietary fiber per day.

Another general diet tip is to choose meals and snacks that are balanced in the three macronutrients. If you've been eating a typical American diet, it's probably carb-heavy. To achieve a better balance, all you need to do is trade some of your carbs for protein and/or fat. For instance, rather than have a whole bagel, spread some peanut butter on half of the bagel and save the other half for later. Rather than have a huge plate of pasta, go for a stir-fry with chicken, vegetables, and a small amount of noodles or rice. A nutrition consultation should go a long way toward helping you find the way of eating that suits you best and keeps you energetic and healthy while helping you change your physique for the better. Some personal trainers offer nutritional and dietary services that are catered to your exercise program and your goals. A registered dietician will be able to provide general nutrition advice for health, weight management, and disease prevention. If you choose to go this route, look for an RD that specializes in weight management or sports nutrition to help you with your fitness goals.

As long as you follow a balanced diet plan that allows you to lose weight in a slow but steady fashion, there are really just two potential problems you might encounter while trying to stick to your diet. One is due to lack of preparation, meaning that you find yourself running out or without access to the foods you need. I address this issue in Reference A. The other potential problem when trying to adhere to your diet plan is dealing with those pesky food cravings.

Food Cravings

If you are like most people, when you feel the urge to overeat or have a food that's not part of your diet plan, an intense urge washes over you. This uncomfortable sensation is what can lead you to abandon your long-term aspirations in exchange for a dose of short-term gratification. If you break a diet that you've already consciously decided is worth following, it's because you were "triggered." The trigger can be internal (feeling low-energy or experiencing a craving) or external (something you see or smell, or a comment from another person). Once you're triggered, you enter into a state of tremendous urgency (7).

Many times having a sense of scarcity, either consciously or subconsciously, is the primary cause of this urgency. You panic because you feel you are being deprived of what you want most of all, and your mind and body are protesting because (consciously or subconsciously) you're worried that you may never get to have the foods you love again. However, while you *think* what you want is the food, what you really want is *to change the way you feel*. You feel deprived because you're not allowing yourself to have the food, which you *know* will change the way you feel, fast (at least for a few moments). You can choose to bypass the food and change the way you feel some other way only if you are able to unlock the stranglehold that the sense of urgency has on you. That's the only way you'll be able to say no for long enough to stop *reacting* and think for a moment about what's really going on.

It's really not tricky at all to stay on track once you learn the basics of "urge management." In assignment 3 of this Strategy I'll explain how to use a tool that can help you get out of that state of urgency. This "urge management tool" will enable you to regain control so you can make better choices – ones that are more conducive to your goals.

Now, as much as I'd love to be able to take credit for coming up with this idea, I learned how to use it through the audiotape "Using Quantity Qualifiers to Change Your Life," which is part of Anthony Robbins' PowerTalk Series. The full bibliographical information can be found in the Notes section in the back of this book (7).

Before you get started learning to control your sense of urgency, you must realize that you're going to feel it anytime something outside of your conscious control triggers you (either involving an internal feeling or an external force). If you use techniques to reduce the intensity of your urgency, you will find your control coming back. Once you have regained control you will be better equipped to break the patterns that can lead you astray, making choices you come to regret.

This technique you are about to learn is an "urge management tool." I will teach you in detail how to use it with food, but you will also be able to apply it to other areas of your life once you understand and practice it. The only way to completely understand how this tool works is to *feel* it in action. I'd like you to turn to part 3 of this Strategy's assignment so you can start experimenting with this tool. Go ahead and complete that assignment before you read any further.

Now I'd like to consider the exercise component of fitness as it relates to "short-term sacrifice." Some people consider exercise a sacrifice that needs to be made in the short-term in order to get what you want in the long-term. It's true that exercise isn't always fun and there are probably a hundred things you'd rather be doing. However, be aware that there are specific workout techniques that allow you to get the most "bang" for your time and effort "buck." In other words, there are ways to become more efficient with your workouts. I like to use the phrase, "work out smarter, not harder for best results." It's true – working out hard is fine and dandy, but if what you're doing doesn't make much physiological sense, you're just wasting your time and energy. Please don't mistake me here – there *will* always be effort required, and don't let those infomercials convince you otherwise. You just want to make sure that you know where and when it's worthwhile to push harder in order to achieve optimal results. You also need to know when to take it easier during your workouts and when you are better served to take a complete break.

For example, consider the person who doesn't know that muscles actually grow while they are resting, not while they are being exercised. Let's suppose that this person trains his chest by performing the bench press every day for a month. This unfortunate (although certainly ambitious) individual will be lucky if his muscles undergo any growth at all. Most likely he will walk away with an overuse injury instead of bigger muscles (assuming he is not taking steroids or the "andro" prohormones, which are precursors to testosterone and allow you to recover faster from workouts).

This person is putting many hours into working his chest, but he would actually see better results if he performed the bench press and other direct chest work just two or three times a week. This would allow his muscles sufficient time to recover before he "breaks them down" again with the weightlifting. See, lifting weights actually creates small tears in the muscle fibers, which is what I mean when I say it "breaks them down." Only when you leave the muscle fibers alone for 36-48 hours will they grow back stronger. Resistance training, then, is one instance where you can get better results with less effort at times.

Another instance where less can mean more for your fitness is seen with building up your cardio endurance. Your endurance will improve faster when you don't work right at your limit during cardio. See, endurance relies on the aerobic or oxygen-using system. If you push yourself too hard during cardio, at some point your body will start working anaerobically, which basically means it uses carbs as fuel because oxygen can't be supplied fast enough to allow your body to burn fat during the activity. While working anaerobically burns lots of calories and therefore promotes the loss of bodyfat, that type of exercise does nothing to increase the efficiency of your aerobic system. Besides the benefit to heart health, what's the benefit of increasing the efficiency of your aerobic system if you can burn calories and lose bodyfat without it?

Well, cardio burns calories too and is one of the best tools you have to create the calorie deficit that is required for you to lose bodyfat. That's because, if you develop your aerobic system, you will be able to go faster for longer than you ever could working anaerobically. This means, in addition to your anaerobic weight-training workouts and your interval training, you will be capable of performing a good amount of steady-pace cardio. Developing the capacity to go faster for longer during cardio means you will be able to burn more calories (which will be calories burned in addition to the calories you burn during resistance training). And you won't develop that capacity if you push yourself *too* much during cardio – that will just trigger your anaerobic system to take over, and your cardiovascular system will fail to adapt for the better. You can't use your anaerobic system for more than 90 seconds at a time, so by definition when you work anaerobically you won't be able to burn as many calories as you can working aerobically (because you'll have to keep stopping when you're working anaerobically – you can only sustain anaerobic work for 60-90 seconds at a time, and you'll also be limited by the amount of carbs stored in your body).

The advice, then, for cardio training is to increase your time and intensity gradually, and only to the pace that you feel you could continue for quite some time if you had to. Speed workouts (where you push yourself as hard as you can for short periods of time) and interval training certainly have their place in fitness, but the primary benefit they provide is fat loss in the short-term – they will only improve your endurance indirectly. And of all the types of exercise, endurance cardio has the potential to burn the greatest number of extra calories during a given week because you can do endurance cardio workouts more often and for longer periods of time without burning out as easily as you'd tend to with the more intense, anaerobic interval training.

I want to make sure that the difference between the two types of training is clear. When you are doing speed workouts or interval training, if your goal is maximum fat loss you *do* want to be sure to push as hard as you can during the "sprints," whether you're cycling, climbing stairs, or running. However, you still need to use your effort judiciously – you need to slow it down during the slower or "recovery" portion of the interval training in order to be able to exert at the level required during the sprints to burn a greater number of calories and trigger the post-exercise calorie burn. Also, you need to space these intense training sessions a few days apart, meaning you should do two per week at the most. That's why you'll still want to optimize your aerobic system – if you do, you'll be able to supplement your weight training and your interval sprints with endurance cardio for a three-pronged approach to fat loss through exercise.

People who can't resist the lure of instant gratification go wrong in different ways. Some will skip their training sessions for more pleasurable activities (they want *instant* pleasure), while others will overdo it by working out too hard or too much (because they want *instant* results) and run themselves into the ground, literally. It's the magic area in between called *moderation* that will get you the best results, particularly in the long-term.

Short-Term Sacrifice assignment

1. Make sure you know how to work out most efficiently to achieve your specific goals. Keep in mind that what's best for you might be different from what's best for someone else, even if you share the same goals. For a starting point, take a look at the tables in Reference D where you'll find workout recommendations based on body type. A trainer should be able to help you become more efficient with your workouts. A few sessions with a trainer can go a long way toward helping you nail down the best approach. To make your workouts more enjoyable, consider buddying up with a workout partner, hiring a trainer, or taking a group exercise class. Even listening to a good CD on your headset or reading a magazine during cardio can make your exercise session something to look forward to.

2. You need to stay focused on what's important to you in the long-term even though your impulses will steer you toward seeking short-term gratification. Take the time to remind yourself that you are an evolved human being who is on a mission to achieve a long-term goal, and you are *willing and able* to sacrifice in the short-term so that you can reach it. Many before you have done so, and you certainly can too. Make sure you understand that fat loss and/or muscle gain aren't going to happen overnight. These changes are the result of a series of behaviors, namely eating the proper amounts of healthy food and working out on a regular basis. You need to give yourself *instant* reinforcement for performing these behaviors on a daily basis if you wish to sustain them, because the final reward won't be realized right away. Just try not to use junk food for your reward! Check to make sure that the points system you've developed for yourself reinforces the behaviors you'll need to perform in order to reach your goals.

Another tip is to track progress in a variety of ways rather than just look at your bodyweight or the amount of weight you can lift at the gym. This is helpful for motivation because sometimes your weight on the scale or your strength in the gym won't change right away even though your body *is* responding to the work you're doing.

Bodyfat percentage is one useful measurement – when you multiply this number by your weight, you will know the amount of bodyfat and the amount of lean tissue you have. If your bodyfat percentage drops, it means that you lost fat and/or gained muscle. If your goal is to tone up and your bodyfat percentage drops, you're right on track. Reaching your ideal weight on the scale will take care of itself in time as long as you're eating right and exercising. Also, keep in mind that a pound of muscle only takes up 60% as much space as a pound of fat, which means you'll be getting smaller and becoming more toned as you build muscle and lose bodyfat. Measure the inches around your waist, hips, and thighs and monitor the way your clothes fit for further indicators of progress or a lack thereof.

Although you can try to take your own measurements, it's best to have someone else take them for accuracy's sake. If you haven't been trained in the proper technique for using bodyfat calipers you won't know how to use them correctly, and there are some areas that you won't be able to reach to measure yourself. It is preferable to have the same person take your measurements each time in order to maintain as much consistency as possible.

Bodyfat scales and handheld bodyfat-reading devices are not the must accurate way to measure your bodyfat percentage. Most of these machines use bioimpedance technology, which means that the device sends a weak electrical current through your body. The time it takes for the current to return to the device correlates with the percentage of lean tissue and percentage of fat in the body. Although these electronic devices aren't as accurate as calipers for finding your true bodyfat percentage, they *are* accurate in measuring trends as long as you're careful to take the measurements during the same time of day and in the same physical state (first thing in the morning is usually the most consistent time). Dehydration, water retention, stored glycogen, and food in your digestive system are just some of the many factors that can skew the measurement. Since there are so many things that can throw off the reading, sometimes it takes a few months' worth of readings to be able to see what's really going on. What's nice about these devices, however, is that you can use them to take your own measurements whenever you'd like.

Although not as sophisticated, a pair of jeans usually works well as a gauge for how you're doing, and the way you look in the mirror is always a good measure of progress, although some people have a hard time seeing positive changes in their body. Ironically, these seem to be the same people who are *very good* at seeing negative things about themselves! Improvements in strength or endurance during your workouts as well as finding that the same workout starts to feel easier are all signs that your fitness is improving and physique changes should be soon to follow. If your workout is spot-on and your physique isn't tightening up much, most likely the culprit is your diet and you'll need to make some changes there in order to see significant changes in your appearance.

3. Now I will cover the "urge management tool" I mentioned in this Strategy. To learn to use the urge management tool, the first thing you need to do is think of a food that you like very much. You'll need to actually go get that food and put it right in front of you before you proceed with this assignment.

Once you have the food in front of you, try to quantify your desire for this particular food on a scale of -10 (completely repulsive) to 0 (neutral; don't really care either way whether or not you have it) to 10 (the most delicious thing ever). This number, even for a given food, will vary at times depending on how long it's been since you've had it, how hungry you are, and other factors. You need to note where you are *right now* on the desire scale, even if you're usually at a different number when thinking about that particular food.

Once you decide where you are on the desire scale, I would like you consciously manipulate your level of desire for this food. For instance, let's say that the food you chose is a chocolate chip cookie and your desire for it is +5. Now you need to ask yourself this question: What would you need to do to bring your desire to +8? Maybe you would need the cookie to be warm. Maybe you would have to imagine that you hadn't had a cookie in years, or that it was one of your mom's homemade cookies.

Whatever does the trick for you, feel your desire moving up to +8. Now you need to figure out what it would take to bring your desire +10. Maybe having milk to dunk it in?

Once you find something that works to increase your desire that much, feel yourself at +10. You've really got to stop, close your eyes, and try this exercise until you are sure you can *feel* your desire at +10. This tool won't work for you in the heat of the moment when you have a craving unless you develop the confidence now that you *do* have control over your urge.

Now that you know you are capable of increasing your desire or your sense of urgency to have the food, you are ready to move forward. You probably achieved an increase in desire by using one of several of different tactics. The most common tactics are:

1. Changing something about the situation.
2. Adding something to the situation
3. Removing a negative consequence from the situation (Would you enjoy the cookie more if you knew it wouldn't lead to weight gain?)

Which of these mechanisms (changing something, adding something, or taking away a negative consequence) did you use to increase your desire?

Now I would like you to practice *decreasing* your desire and urgency. This is the tool that will really come in handy when you're trying to stick to your diet – I know, that last exercise seemed like I was trying to sabotage you! One way to decrease urgency is simply to break the pattern. Have you ever had a craving and then been distracted by something else, only to find that when you thought of the food again you weren't craving it so badly anymore? Changing your focus away from the craving takes the intensity away in many cases (it takes the edge off).

Diversion, or changing focus, is one method you can use to dodge cravings. While there are three primary tactics you can use to increase or decrease desire, changing focus is a fourth tactic that is primarily used to decrease desire.

If you choose to stay focused on the craving or can't find a way to divert yourself, you might decide to consciously lower your desire for the food by changing something about the situation or adding something to the situation (tactics 1 and 2 from the list on the last page), and for the purpose of decreasing urgency you'll be changing something from good to bad or adding something negative. Using the cookie example, you might imagine that you've added something that doesn't taste good to the cookie. Imagine eating it then – yeck! Some people go as far as to picture it moldy or spoiled, or they imagine themselves so stuffed that no food, no matter how tasty, sounds good. Bring yourself all the way down to -10 on the desire scale using whatever thought or tactic it takes.

Thinking of the health and weight consequences works to decrease desire for junk food in some people (tactic 3 from the list – but instead of *taking away* a negative consequence like you'd do to increase desire, you'd *emphasize* it to decrease desire), but this "intellectual" knowledge usually isn't as powerful as actually making yourself feel "grossed out" by the food, because being "grossed out" keeps you from wanting it at all. It takes "willpower" out of the equation completely. This is important because no matter what you tell yourself *intellectually* regarding how bad the food is for you, as a human being you are still wired to go after the short-term pleasure of eating in spite of the fact that it means long-term pain. However, if you can eliminate the short-term pleasure associated with the food, not wanting it will become very easy.

Find which method works best to decrease desire for the food you have in front of you. Be sure to stay with these exercises until you are sure that you *feel* the changes in your body (not just think, but *feel*) as you move toward reaching the point where you don't even want the food anymore. It's only once you are able to experience that change in feeling that you will be confident you have the ability to keep your urges under control.

See, for almost everyone, just thinking about how you don't want to eat the food won't be enough. I know in the past you've probably thought about how bad a certain food was for you, decided that you didn't want it, and then went ahead and ate it anyway. This process I'm teaching you is different because I'm teaching you how to actually stop desiring it in the first place. That is very different from intellectually knowing it isn't good for you but still craving the food in spite of that fact. When you feel tortured by cravings you're not in control – you're subject to whatever your environment throws at you. If you don't have a plan to help you stay focused on what you really want for your life, you'll be subject to the whims of others who might be oblivious to the harm they could be causing you, or might even be strategically acting to influence you to their advantage. Marketers prey on this kind of thing. They make more and more money every time you make an impulse decision. Even your friends benefit in some cases when they encourage you to overeat, drink too much, or have junk food. If you partake, they don't feel so bad about doing it themselves. We use social comparisons to justify many of our behaviors that we know deep down aren't right. That's why people who engage in harmful behaviors tend to surround themselves with others who do the same thing. It's easier to tell ourselves that something is okay if other people are doing it, too.

Once you've improved your urge management skills, exercising "discipline" will be so much easier. If you develop the ability to control the way you feel, *you can actually obliterate the craving from the inside out.* If you become really good at this, you literally won't even *want* the food anymore. You will actually teach yourself to be disgusted by it. *Although other people will say that you're so "disciplined," you'll secretly know that you're not even tempted anymore.* Having this ability will infuse you with incredible power because you'll know that you're always capable of "taking back the reins" in the face of any trigger. The environment is full of triggers that have the potential to influence the way you act. You can be one step ahead of things simply by being aware of this phenomenon. You will benefit so much once you develop the ability to change the way you feel on your own, without having to use food or any other substance to affect this change. The main reason people are motivated to perform any action or behavior is that they want to change the way they feel, either now or in the future. Once you are able to accomplish this using techniques in your own mind, you won't have to resort to doing anything that works against your goals.

And, once you've been avoiding certain foods for a few weeks, you will find that it gets easier and easier to say no because you will have broken the habit. At that point, you might not even need to go through the process of bringing yourself down on the desire scale in order to regain control. However, once you've learned how to use this urge management tool, you'll always have it at your disposal in case you need it. Just the idea of having it available to you at all times should go a long way toward helping you stay on track.

After completing this assignment, please go back to the reading on page 158.

4. When dealing with food cravings, the urge management tool is quite useful for decreasing your sense of urgency to eat things that will hinder your progress. However, you can also use the urge management tool to *increase* your sense of urgency or desire where you need it – for instance, you can use it to increase your want to exercise or to develop the capacity to fully enjoy *anything* you do, even something that isn't typically perceived as a pleasurable activity.

The first step in applying the urge management tool to other areas of your life is to refer back to the pattern that you used to increase your desire for a particular food. Remember, the three tactics are: changing something about the situation, adding something to the situation, or removing a negative consequence. Whichever worked for you, try applying that approach to other areas of your life besides food cravings.

For instance, think back to the cookie example. If you added something pleasant to the cookies to make them seem more desirable, such as milk to dunk them in, try using that pattern (the pattern of adding something) in another area of your life where you'd like to increase desire. If you're trying to increase your desire to exercise, think of what you can do to make the experience of exercising more pleasant. Perhaps this could involve listening to music you like, or reading a good magazine while you're on the cardio equipment. Maybe it could be going to the gym with your significant other or your best friend.

Look to various aspects of your life and find areas where you'd benefit by either increasing or decreasing desire. Then try to manipulate your level of desire by applying the patterns that worked for you in the cookie example. If you develop the ability to manipulate your desire, you'll be able to affect a change in almost any area of your life easily and permanently. Also, you'll find that, once you realize you *do* have control over your feelings, you'll be able to make more things in your life a "must" instead of just a "should." If you have the attitude "I must" go to the gym, you will go much more often than you will if it is only a "should" for you.

Don't believe me? Let's see what you currently categorize as a "must" and what is currently just a "should" for you. Hopefully, you have the belief that you "must" pay your bills. What if that was just a "should" for you? Would you find yourself in trouble? Things become automatic when they are a "must." You waste less time worrying, procrastinating, and coming up with excuses. Instead, you get right to doing what you need to do.

Making exercise a "must" only requires two specific abilities: You need to be able to maintain control of your feelings while exercising, and you need to have several options available for getting your exercise.

You'll find that you are able to raise your personal standards as you learn to ask the right questions of yourself, such as, "What do I need to do to feel the way I want to feel?" From now on, always know that you have the urge management tool at your disposal, because if you don't make it a point to take control of your life, the world won't hesitate to take control of you!

Strategy 16: Really *Needing* it

How to make success a necessity in your life

If you think back over your life up until now, you'll probably be able to come up with a list of achievements that hold some significance for you. If you don't mind settling for what you have already achieved, you don't need to worry about pushing yourself any further. However, if you don't want to stop growing as a person, (and if you *do* stop, that's almost a surefire way to a boring, unfulfilling life) the first thing you need to do is take inventory of all the abilities you possess. The second thing you need to do is ask yourself this question: "Who wants to have a great life with just a few pieces missing in the puzzle?"

No matter what you have accomplished and what titles you hold, you'll never feel completely satisfied and happy until you have your health under control, which includes not only feeling great, but looking great too. Once you acknowledge this, you should feel hungry to make more out of your life, and achieving success in all areas will become a necessity for you. You really can "have it all" as long as you're willing to keep learning and keep putting an effort out there, and as long as you're willing to balance your life across many areas.

The other point you must remember is that, as a young person, you can sometimes skate by and stay relatively fit and healthy without having to do much to maintain it. The older you get, the further you will slip from your physical ideal *unless you exercise regularly and eat well.* Therefore, by not working on your health and fitness you are actually *decreasing* your standing in that area – you're not even holding steady. Observing this trend in action is how the myth that you lose muscle and body tone as you age came about. Some people are able to maintain great looks in their youth no matter what they do or don't do, but on some level *everyone* falls prey to the repercussions of living an inactive, unhealthy lifestyle as they age. So, you really have two choices – you can either let yourself slide, or you can decide to improve yourself with proper nutrition and exercise. If you let yourself slide, sooner or later nothing else in life will matter much because you will look and feel exactly the way you've been treating your body all these years, and it sure won't be pretty.

It's also a fact that the younger you are and the less out-of-shape you are, the easier it will be to make amends and get yourself back in shape. It's *twice as hard* to get into shape as it is to simply maintain what you've got. If you put the effort in now, you can nip any problems in the bud, saving yourself a lot of hard work in the future. You can't change the unhealthy lifestyle you might have led in the past, but you *can* make up your mind to change now, because it sure won't get any easier the longer you wait to get started.

Really *Needing* it assignment

1. Ask yourself the question, "What have I already achieved in my life?" Make two columns on the next fresh page in your notebook. List these past and present achievements, along with the character traits you possess that led to your success in each endeavor. If you had the strength to do those things, don't you have the strength to improve your health and fitness too? Hopefully your answer to that question is "yes"– and you can use this confirmation to help bolster your belief that you *do* have what it takes to get what you want out of life.

Many people deny that they have a need to achieve success in a certain area, not because they don't want it, but because they don't want to be disappointed if they fail. They'd rather not try than risk disappointing themselves. However, I invite you to look at the situation logically: When you take information contained in this book and combine that with the obvious abilities and character that you've already proven you have, what could possibly stop you from achieving anything at all once you decide that you *really need it*?

Strategy 17: Just do *something*

How exercise action and mini-workouts yield results

Especially when you're first starting an exercise program, consistency is the most important aspect of your training. As a beginner, the most important issue is the number of days per week that you train. This means, if something prevents you from completing your full session (a full session for you might be anything from 10 minutes to an hour), you need to commit to doing at least some percentage of that. No matter what it takes, you've got to find a way to fit it into your day. You might have to get creative and it might not be easy, but think about it this way – if someone would pay you a million dollars to do it, would you be able to find a way? We're talking 5 or 10 minutes here.

See, there is a point of diminishing returns with exercise. Just doing any at all gives you so much benefit. In fact, for beginners, the first 10-15 minutes of a well-designed exercise program yields about 50% of the benefit you'd get out of a 60-minute session. For intermediate and advanced exercisers, the same holds true as long as you boost your intensity during that shorter time frame.

I'll give you an example of the thinking process to go through when you're crunched for time. Let's assume that an unexpected project comes up at work that cannot be put off. This leaves you with only 20 minutes to work out (and we'll assume that you normally exercise for 45 minutes). To make matters worse, even though you usually work out at the gym, you realize that you aren't going to have time to get there. No problem – you can simply do an abbreviated workout at home.

If you're doing a short workout, you'll get better results if you increase your intensity by lifting more weight and/or reduce the amount of time spent resting between sets (this applies mostly to intermediate and advanced exercisers, since beginners just need to focus on being consistent with the number of days per week they work out). Do your best to produce a similar effect on your body as you would get from your regular workout. For instance, if you had intended to work your chest using free weights, try push-ups at home for an alternative.

I'll give you a sample chest, shoulder and triceps routine that doesn't take long to do and can be done at home. All sets should be done close to muscular failure, and anything from 5-25 reps is fine – do as many reps per set as you can get with good form. The workout is listed on the next page. If you are unsure of the correct form for a push-up, turn to Reference C under the section "Fit with Four" for instructions on how to do push-ups and pictures of the correct form.

Chest, shoulder, and triceps home workout

1. Do a set of decline push-ups with your knees or toes on the edge of a couch and your hands on the floor. Rest 30-60 seconds.
2. Do a set of regular push-ups on the floor off your knees (easier) or off your toes (more advanced). Rest 30-60 seconds.
3. Do a set of incline push-ups with your knees or toes on the floor and your hands on the edge of a couch. Rest 30-60 seconds.

Repeat this sequence three times and you just might get a better workout than you've been getting at the gym! During a resistance-training workout targeting the chest, shoulders, and triceps, a traditional workout involves some compound exercises (like the bench press and dumbbell chest press) followed by some isolation exercises (like the dumbbell fly for chest, the lateral raise for shoulders, and the cable pushdown for triceps). You'd typically work in the 6-12-rep range and rest for a minute or two between sets to accommodate the relatively heavy weights that result in muscular fatigue by 6-12 reps.

But isn't the traditional workout better, you ask? Not necessarily. It's just *different* – not better or worse. The best overall resistance-training program includes weightlifting *and* bodyweight exercises (meaning you move your own bodyweight for resistance). The best overall program also utilizes various lengths of rest periods between sets, at times taking no rest between sets and at times taking up to 5 minutes of rest between sets. So, you're really not missing out on anything when you do the abbreviated home routine. Even if you had all the time in the world, I would still recommend using a wide range of workout types, lengths, and intensities.

If you wanted to incorporate some cardio into the "push-up workout" outlined above, you could do jumping jacks, jump rope, aerobic stepping, or marching in place for 60-90 seconds between your sets of push-ups.

What if you had been planning for a long session at the gym? In that case you'll probably need to do a substitute workout on the day you are squeezed for time, and switch your long workout to another day. No big deal.

If you wanted to focus on cardio for that shorter workout session, try a combination of moves such as jumping jacks, running in place, stair climbing, and bodyweight-only jump-squats. Spend 30-90 seconds on each, and repeat until you've completed at least five minutes of cardio, continuing for up to 30 minutes if you have the time and the stamina. This routine should get you pretty winded and will definitely blast some calories and fat. Jumping rope all by itself is perfect for a short but intense cardio session – and the same goes for jogging, walking hills, stair-climbing, or aerobic stepping at home.

I know these "mini-workouts" might be a little tougher than the workouts you're used to. What should you do if you wanted to shorten a planned workout not because of a time crunch, but because of an energy crunch? If fatigue or exhaustion is the problem and you aren't motivated to tackle a full-length session, you probably won't be up for increasing your intensity even if it's just for 10 or 15 minutes. However, doing *anything at all* fitness-wise for any length of time will at least keep you on track with your commitment, plus it will burn some calories, elevate your mood and energy level, and boost your metabolism for the day. A walk or a few sets of resistance movements like no-added-weight squats and push-ups against a wall make for a great mini-workout when you are operating at less than full speed.

Another reason you should try to do something even when you don't feel up for it is that feeling tired or unmotivated does not necessarily mean that you'll have a poor workout or you'll struggle to get through the session. Exercise is a mood-booster and an energy-booster. Sometimes you won't feel like working out because you have had a stressful or boring day and you feel drained or lethargic. In these cases, exercise is probably just what you need to feel better. For times when you just don't feel like working out, I recommend starting your workout but taking it easy for the first ten or fifteen minutes. Don't feel obligated to do your entire workout just because you started – wait and see how you feel after about fifteen minutes. If you still aren't into it, you might be wasting your time if you force yourself to continue. However, your endorphins (the "feel-good" hormones) should start kicking in after about the 15-minute mark, which might lift your mood and make you want to keep going. Mood and energy level beforehand have very little to do with the quality of workout you will have, so give yourself a chance even if you don't feel like working out.

Just do *something* assignment

1. Read through Reference C, "Just How Much Time is Required to Experience the Benefits of Exercise?" Also, review the descriptions of the basic exercises that make up "Fit with Four." Learn and practice the moves when you're not pressed for time so that when you *are*, you'll have an effective workout option.

2. If you aren't comfortable with the exercises described, consult a trainer. After you know how to do these fundamental exercises, you'll be well on your way to mastering the basics of resistance training. Whether you're male or female, young or old, and experienced or inexperienced with exercise, you can use these moves your entire life to maintain your looks, your strength, and your health. Everyone from an elderly person hoping to maintain quality of life to a bodybuilder competing for the world championship has a use for these four basic movements in his exercise routine and will see continual progress and results from performing them.

Strategy 18: Time on your side

How to make the time to be a regular exerciser

Lack of time is the number-one excuse people give for why they don't exercise regularly. Although I can sympathize with being busy, it's a big misconception that exercise has to take a lot of time. Of course, some people have such poor time management skills that they don't seem to have *any* time to spare. Time management is an important issue, and I'll be sure to address it in this Strategy and assignment.

The amount of time you should take for exercise depends on your goals. You need to decide what you'd like to get out of your exercise program. If you're like most people you are thinking about adopting an exercise program because you want to look and feel better. To accomplish these objectives, you need to perform movements that exercise and strengthen all the muscles in your body (resistance training) including the heart muscle (cardio). Many people also exercise to help control their weight.

All of these objectives can be achieved most *efficiently* with a circuit-training program. Circuit training isn't the best type of training to use all the time if you're looking for top-notch results, but it is by far the most efficient way to get in good shape. For someone who isn't going to spend more than 1-3 hours a week on exercise or who simply wants to get the most bang for his buck while exercising, it's the best compromise.

A circuit-training program is a resistance-training program where you perform one exercise after another without resting between sets and then complete the "loop" of exercises a few more times (the exact number of exercises and loops depends on your goals and the length of your exercise session). Another option for circuit training is to pick two exercises that don't use the same muscle groups and alternate between the two until you've completed all your sets for those exercises before moving on to another two exercises. The key for both types of circuit training is to avoid standing around between sets – at any given time you should be either doing an exercise or else moving as quickly as possible to the next one. Circuit training elevates your heart rate and, as long as you keep moving, should keep it elevated for the majority of the session, which means that circuit training provides many of the benefits of cardiovascular exercise. Of course, the cardiovascular benefit is in addition to the strength increase and boost in metabolism you get from the resistance training.

If you perform circuit training and watch your diet *closely*, you shouldn't need to do any cardio sessions in order to lose weight and tone up. This will allow you to drastically cut down on total workout time per week. Cardio is, after all, the most time-consuming aspect of working out. The cardio component of your workout (which has the purpose of burning calories, building endurance and working the heart muscle) can be covered more or less by moving quickly from one exercise to the next during your resistance training. In an ideal world you would make more time for workouts, but by using circuit training you can accomplish the most for your fitness in the least amount of time.

On the other hand, if you choose to do cardio but try to save time by skipping resistance training, you will find it harder to reduce your bodyfat in the long run. This is because you'll eventually lose muscle (studies show this occurs after about four weeks being away from resistance training), and your metabolism will drop as a result. When it comes to muscle mass, if you don't use it you lose it! Even cardiovascular activities that use the lower body such as running or climbing stairs won't condition your leg muscles the same way that resistance training will.

Many times the muscle loss will happen slowly when you neglect resistance training, but it creeps up on you to the tune of, on average, a 1-pound gain in bodyfat per year and a 1-pound loss of muscle mass per year, even if your total bodyweight stays the same. Of course, if your weight on the scale goes up, more likely than not you've put on even more bodyfat. Keep in mind, too, that a pound of muscle takes up only 60% as much space as a pound of fat. To be exact, a pound of fat has 1.7 times the volume of a pound of muscle (2). What does that mean for your appearance? If you stay at the same weight but have lost muscle and gained fat, you will be bigger, not to mention looser and more "flabby." You might still fit into your clothes the first few years this happens, but sooner or later you'll notice that your clothes are significantly tighter. Up until that point you'll *think* everything is fine since your weight stayed the same.

Since muscle burns calories and fat does not, every year that you lose muscle and gain fat you will burn fewer calories. Having a slower metabolism means that eventually you will start gaining weight on the scale, even if you eat exactly the same way. *This "sudden" weight gain was not really sudden at all – it was actually years in-the-making.* You might claim (and honestly believe) that you "suddenly" gained weight once you hit a certain age. Usually, the culprit isn't age – rather, it's the gradual loss of muscle tissue and the gradual increase in fat mass over the years, which results in a slower metabolism. All of a sudden your body takes up more space and your weight starts to climb. Your clothes feel snug, especially in places like the hips, thighs, and stomach (women) and all around the waistline including the low back (men), and it happens quickly because each year you have been burning fewer and fewer calories per day, and that's bound to catch up to you at some point.

Obviously something needs to be done about this situation, but many people are hesitant to start working out because they feel that they're already too busy as it is. You know that you can make the time for anything that is really important to you, so if you decide that working out is important for your success and happiness you will be able to make the time. You'll be happy to know that you don't have to spend much time on workouts to benefit from exercise. If you don't have very much free time, you'll want to get the most bang for your buck when you take the time to work out. You can think of working out with *weights* as an investment in your metabolism for the future, on top of the calorie burn you will get today from the exercise.

Cardio has the potential to burn calories faster than resistance training if you do an intense workout, but the benefits of cardio for weight loss are short-lived. You burned the calories today, but you have to do it again and again to see that same calorie burn in the future. Any day you don't do the cardio is a day that you won't burn those extra calories. Also, too much cardio actually lowers your basal metabolic rate (BMR) over time as your body, feeling threatened by the high energy expenditure, downgrades your metabolism to conserve energy.

On the other hand, when you focus on resistance training as a means to build muscle, you burn more calories every day whether you exercise or not. Also, you can maintain the muscle you've built (and the high metabolism that goes along with it) with less frequent and less intense workouts than it took to build the muscle. You only need to train a particular muscle once per week to maintain what you've got. Also, remember that it takes about one month to lose significant amounts of muscle mass once you stop training, but for that entire month you will continue to benefit from the elevated metabolism (compare that to the daily cardio workouts that are required if you want to continue to burn the extra calories every day). You will still continue to benefit from the muscle mass you built during resistance training after you've been away from it for over a month, but the extra calorie burn will grow smaller and smaller the more muscle you lose. On the contrary, if you stop following your cardio routine, starting that very day you won't burn any more calories than you would if you had never trained at all.

There's even more good news about resistance training. Muscles have what's commonly known as "muscle memory," which means you can rapidly regain strength levels that dropped off when you stopped training with weights for whatever reason. You might feel weak as a kitten your first day back, but you will be shocked by how quickly your strength and your muscle mass return. Assuming you never had huge muscles to begin with, you can regain virtually all your strength and muscle tissue more quickly than you can your cardiovascular level after you've taken some time off. The reason is that cardiovascular endurance improves the fastest when you work at a moderate level and are consistent with it, so you won't be able to hasten your return to cardiovascular fitness like you can with resistance training.

Just when you think the benefits of resistance training can't get any better, listen to this: Besides the future payoff you get when you perform resistance training, it also cranks up your post-workout calorie expenditure provided that you work out with a sufficient amount of tension, or weight. This bonus is partly due to the workout intensity and the type of fuel used for resistance training (it's anaerobic, or carbohydrate/non-oxygen using, work) and partly due to the energy-intensive muscle rebuilding process that occurs following a resistance-training session. When you perform cardio, you burn calories during the session but don't typically see a significant boost in metabolic rate following the session. Interval sprints at a near-maximum heart rate can lead to the post-workout calorie burn, but if you're slightly out-of-shape or overweight you aren't going to be able to complete these safely, whereas it's more likely that you'll be able to get through an intense resistance training workout. Besides, interval sprints aren't really "cardio" per se because they are an anaerobic activity. They *are* a great way to burn calories though, which is why some people use them as a substitute for cardio in their exercise routine to burn calories faster.

So, if we're talking about weight loss, cardio has a clear but limited benefit. Sure, it burns calories, but it takes a long time to burn off a significant number of calories during cardio. In fact, to lose weight as a direct result of walking or running you'd have to log about 35 miles to lose one pound! Any amount of cardio beyond three 20-minute sessions a week won't give you much in the way of additional fat loss beyond what you could have achieved simply by eating fewer calories. Of course, if you have a hard time keeping your calorie intake down, cardio can be of help because it burns extra calories. Unfortunately, though, calories can be consumed much faster than they can be burned! However, if you have the time, doing at least a light cardio session every day will increase the calories-out side of your metabolic equation, meaning you will be able to eat a little more and hopefully still run a sufficient calorie deficit to lose weight. Just be careful when using this logic to allow yourself to eat more, because the average person is lucky to burn 400-500 calories during an hour of cardio – the amount in a bagel from Dunkin' Donuts with half a serving of the cream cheese. So, obviously you can't eat *too* much more just because you do extra cardio, but you *can* make up for a few hundred calories if you're willing to spend that much time exercising.

I've spent all this time talking about cardio because there are so many misconceptions about its role in weight loss. However, my intention is *not* to downplay the importance of cardiovascular exercise. There are many benefits to cardio, and cardio is definitely worth doing. Cardio does wonders for heart health and long-term weight management when it's performed in conjunction with a resistance-training program. It's just that, especially considering the amount of time it takes, cardio is not a critical component of weight loss like proper diet and resistance training are. I must mention, though, that women in general tend to lose weight more easily when they do cardio, whereas that's not necessarily the case for men. Men can usually lose just fine doing resistance training and watching their diet, especially in the early stages of weight loss. However, if a man isn't keeping a sufficient calorie deficit to lose weight without cardio, adding cardio will definitely help. Cardio also becomes increasingly important the leaner a man gets if he wants to continue losing bodyfat. For all men, a cardio regimen will probably be required to take off the last 5-10 pounds of unwanted bodyfat.

Women tend to need cardio even when their diet is clean, especially when they're trying to lose the last 10-20 pounds of excess bodyfat. One reason more cardio is needed is that women don't burn as many calories as men: As a general rule they are shorter, lighter, and carry less muscle mass at a given weight. They also tend to have slightly slower metabolisms, even when comparing two individuals of the same size. This means that it's harder for women to create a sufficient calorie deficit through diet alone. Also, women don't typically burn as many calories when they lift weights because they generally lift lighter weights than men.

The calorie-burning issue aside, women also carry more of what's categorized as "stubborn fat" on their hips and thighs. This type of fat isn't mobilized easily, but if you increase blood flow to the area it helps with fat mobilization. Cardio is the best way to accomplish this. Men have stubborn fat too, although they usually don't have as much of it as women. The male version of stubborn fat is typically found on the abdomen and isn't quite as difficult to mobilize because there is more blood flow to the abdomen than there is to the hips and thighs. Even so, men wanting to get rid of their stubborn fat deposits will find that cardio usually does the trick.

One interesting thing about cardio is that people who are consistent about their cardiovascular exercise tend to *maintain* their weight quite well. They typically don't gain much weight (if they gain any at all) from year to year, and there's something to be said for simply *not gaining weight*, especially today when obesity runs rampant! However, people who do cardio don't usually *lose* much weight *unless they're also watching their diet*, running a calorie deficit sufficient to allow for weight loss. Cardio can help tip the scales toward a calorie deficit since it burns calories, but it can't make up for a bad diet. In other words, cardio can be a *tool* to help create a calorie deficit, but it won't take off bodyfat *unless* you have a calorie deficit.

If I had my way, everyone would carve out enough time to do at least a couple of cardio and weight training sessions per week, spending up to an hour exercising, 2-3 times per week. But for super-busy people, where to find this time? See this Strategy's assignment for help.

If you want to try a routine that will give you the benefits of cardio and weights but won't take more than 30 minutes, 2-3 times a week, try a beginner's circuit-training workout. Use the four exercises as detailed in Reference C. Perform one set of each, and repeat the entire circuit 3-6 times. This should take 15-30 minutes depending on how many rounds you do, and constitutes a general fitness program that should yield good results when performed 2-3 times per week. Your strength and stamina will definitely go up, and you'll lose bodyfat as well. You'll also lose bodyweight if you need to, as long as your diet is on track.

Worried you'll get behind on other things when you take the time to start working out regularly? Don't! Adding a workout to your schedule tends to make your day more productive overall. In other words, you can work out *and* have more time left for work and play. One reason I say this is because physical fitness has been directly linked to improved work performance (8). It turns out that lifestyle-related health risks have a significant impact on job performance. People who engage in moderate exercise do higher-quality work and demonstrate better job performance than those who lead sedentary lifestyles. Physically fit employees get along better with co-workers and take fewer sick days than out-of-shape employees. It seems that people with better cardiovascular fitness and more strength perform tasks faster and do them with less effort.

Apparently some employers and health organizations are taking note and encouraging their employees to adopt fitness programs. Some companies are providing longer lunch hours to workers who choose to exercise on their lunch break. Some are building or improving office gyms, while others offer discounts or free memberships to fitness clubs or even cash bonuses to employees who work out. As nice as it is to think that employers are just looking out for the well-being of their employees, these changes are occurring primarily because employers are starting to realize the financial benefits of encouraging physical fitness among their workers. Apparently, increasing physical activity to moderate levels is associated with declines in annual health care charges of, on average, $2,000 per employee (8). This savings is a bonus on top of the increased productivity a company enjoys when its workers are physically fit.

Time on your side assignment

1. Open your notebook to the next blank page and answer these questions:

–What do you do that you consider to be a "time waster," meaning that it takes time out of your day without giving you much benefit?
–Do you say "yes" when people ask you to do things, even when you don't really have the extra time? Can you start saying "no" sometimes so that you can take the time to do what is really important for you and your health?
–What task(s) can you delegate to someone else so that you can carve out time to exercise?
–Have you been working through your lunch hour? Do you even *have* a lunch hour? Can you demand that hour for yourself and do your workout then? Can you ask to go into work later so you can squeeze in a morning workout? If not, can you wake up a little earlier so that you can work out? What about evenings? Can you set aside some time two evenings a week and one weekend day for working out?

2. Schedule your exercise like you would any other appointment. Scheduling exercise first thing in the morning works well for many people. In fact, morning exercisers have the best track record for adhering to their fitness programs. If you work out in the morning, it's done and over with while your energy level is still high, and you have a better chance of getting your session in before something else comes up to interfere with your plans. In the early morning, the phone isn't ringing off the hook and there aren't as many distractions. If you work out in the morning, you'll also tend to feel better all day and will be more motivated to stick to your diet.

In spite of all these reasons to exercise in the a.m., you need to pick the time to work out that's best for you. If you're simply *not* a morning person, it doesn't make sense to try to force yourself to exercise at the crack of dawn. No matter what time of day you choose, the key is to make it a nonnegotiable event. With everything that seems to be vying for you attention, you'd be surprised at how many things really can wait. I know people who used to spend a half-hour each day vacuuming the house or doing another similar chore. When they adopted an exercise program, they decided to do that chore only every other day, and on the days they skipped it they exercised instead. They hardly noticed the difference when they vacuumed less, but the difference in their body and the way they felt as a result of the workouts was significant. The point is, you can figure out ways to save 30 minutes here or there.

You will be more energetic and become more productive when you follow a workout program, so make your workouts the last thing you'd ever push aside.

I know people who complain that eating healthy takes too much time. However, many of these people go out to eat on a regular basis and spend one or two hours at the restaurant. Cooking and eating healthy takes just a fraction of that time. Review Reference A, "The 10 Tricks You Need to Know to Eat Right, one person at a time." If you prefer to eat out, there are plenty of healthy options – in fact, you have more choices today than ever before. See the articles "Eating Out the Healthy Way" and "Fast-food on a Diet" in Reference B. You might find it a bit challenging to resist ordering your favorite dish, but if you get yourself in the mindset that you eat healthy even when you eat out, you'll be fine.

Strategy 19: Do it right or don't do it at all

Strict form makes all the difference

If you use correct form on your exercises it literally makes all the difference. An exercise can feel five times harder (and actually be five times more effective) when you use correct form. If you perform an exercise with 40 pounds using improper alignment or using momentum to lift the weight, you'd actually be better off using just 20-30 pounds and doing the exercise the right way. Not only will you develop your muscles better, but you'll also reduce your risk for injury when you do the exercise correctly and don't try to use more weight than you can properly handle.

When you do an exercise right, you'll work the target area more intensely even if you have to use less weight. Your muscles have no clue what number is stamped on the dumbbell you're using – they simply know how hard they're working. That's why you will get better results with lighter weights if you've been "cheating" with the heavier ones.

Making sure you use the right weight and the correct form on an exercise isn't just something that personal trainers do to make you miserable, or to humble you by telling you that you're not strong enough for the heavier weights. Working out with correct form is the safest, most effective, and most efficient way to train. As an intermediate or advanced exerciser, you'll want to vary your lifting speed and your lifting technique for specific reasons at times. However, you can never go wrong by going back to the basics, which include lifting slowly and deliberately instead of using momentum, training in a full range of motion, and keeping the resistance, or tension, focused on the target muscle group.

When you use improper form, whether it's because you're trying to lift a weight that's too heavy or because you simply don't know how to do an exercise correctly, you don't burn as many calories because your joints, rather than your muscles, absorb the brunt of the tension and pressure. Your body burns calories and gets stronger when you use your *muscle tissue*, not when you stress your joints. By using control, keeping the correct form, and lifting a weight you can manage, you'll be able to focus the resistance on your muscles. All you'll get from burdening your joints with more than their fair share of the work is an injury. And if you get injured, you will have to back off from exercise until you've healed. In the worst-case scenario, you might never completely recover from an injury – it can bother you for the rest of your life. It just doesn't pay to use poor form!

Do it right or don't do it at all assignment

1. Turn to Reference C under the subheading "Fit with Four" where you'll find instructions for performing some basic resistance-training exercises and pictures of the correct form. To learn more exercises, hire a trainer or look to the resources listed in Reference E.

2. Make sure that your training routine is balanced. Even if you perform all of your exercises correctly, you will develop muscular imbalances if you work some muscle groups with more volume and/or intensity than others. Always keep tabs on your routine and your form. Also, keep in mind that different workout routines and form techniques might be more appropriate as you progress.

Pay particular attention to the following areas, because the most common form mistakes I see involve:
    a. Making an exercise easier by limiting range-of-motion during an exercise.
    b. Moving too fast, which means using momentum to lift the weight and allowing gravity (instead of your muscles) to lower it.
    c. Doing exercises the right way when reminded, but slowly drifting into bad form over time if no one is monitoring you.

Most people don't do these things on purpose – they *want* to do the exercises right, but they unknowingly start with (or begin slipping into) bad habits. The body will naturally try to take "the path of least resistance" while, ironically, doing resistance training (your body wants to exert the least amount of effort required to complete a task in order to conserve energy and strength – think "survival mechanism"). Don't believe me? When you're carrying something heavy, you will automatically find the easiest way to carry it, which will be the way that uses the least amount of energy and effort. Also, after carrying it for a while you'll shift the object you're holding to your other side or change the way you hold it to avoid taxing one particular muscle group too much. During resistance training, keep in mind that your *goal* is to exert as much effort as possible during a movement and to make *sure* to tax a particular muscle group. If you feel an uncomfortable tension in your muscles while lifting weights, that's a good thing – it means you're applying resistance to your muscles. Instead of trying to find a comfortable way to do the exercise, put your body in the very position that makes the exercise feel the most strenuous for best results.

When reviewing your exercise routine, be aware that the most common mistakes I see in routine design involve:
   a. Doing too many lifts for the "mirror muscles" (chest, abs, biceps, quads, and front head of the shoulder) and not enough for the muscles in the back of the body (back, hamstrings, triceps, and rear head of the shoulder).
   b. Spending too much time on weights and not enough time on cardio, or vice-versa (People tend to do more of what they happen to like, and tend to perform certain types of exercises disproportionately or to the exclusion of others when they buy into a fitness myth).
   c. Sticking with the same program for too long. Your program should be revamped every 6-8 weeks to ensure that you continue progressing at the fastest pace. It also should be modified based on your results from the past month or two, meaning that you'll want to look at your training log and your measurements to gauge how well the program worked. This will provide clues as to what is most likely to work best in the coming months.

Strategy 20: Better safe than sorry

How to exercise to get healthy, not to get injured

Safety needs to be your number-one priority during your workout. Using correct form goes a long way toward helping you stay injury-free. There are certain exercises, however, that will always bother some people, even when they are performed correctly. People who are predisposed to knee or shoulder problems tend to have trouble with certain exercises. You probably won't know which exercises are apt to bother you unless a specialist such as an orthopedic doctor or a physical therapist has warned you to avoid particular movements. Most people don't know which exercises might be troublesome until they actually try them. For example, movements such as lunges and the upright row are good exercises that have their place in everyone's routine, but they tend to cause pain in the joints for some people. Since they are two of the best exercises for their respective target muscle groups, you'll want to do them as long as they don't bother you. You'll need to use trial and error to see if any exercises cause pain for you. It's highly unlikely that you will do permanent damage by trying an exercise as long as you stop at the first sign of pain. A trainer can recommend substitute exercises or help you change your form or the amount of weight used so that the exercise isn't painful to perform.

At times you'll find that the weight you've been using isn't challenging you anymore. When experimenting with a new weight, it's definitely better to be safe than sorry. Increase the amount of weight you use just a little at a time (anything from 2-10 pounds, depending on the lift). You can always do a few more reps if the weight you've chosen hasn't taxed you to the limit, and you'll know to choose a heavier weight next time (since you *do* need to hit muscular fatigue in the 6-12-rep range for best results). What will really set you back, though, is getting hurt and having to rest the injured area while it heals.

All this advice about being careful *doesn't* mean that you should use light weights. You should definitely choose a weight that feels difficult to lift. That's the only way you'll accomplish all the benefits of resistance training that I've been telling you about. If a weight feels heavy in the 5-8-rep range and you don't have pain in the joints while lifting, you should use that weight for some of your workouts. Just make sure to vary your training to include some lighter-weight, higher-rep workouts as well (meaning 6-12 or even 15 reps). Including some lighter-weight workouts will give your joints and muscles adequate time to recover while still helping you maintain your muscle mass and strength. Don't lift super-heavy (in the 3-5-rep range) for the same bodypart more frequently than once per week. If you feel pain at any point during a rep or set, you should take the cue to back off a bit. If this happens, avoid heavy-weight, low-rep sets for the time being and stay with lighter weights and higher reps until you've been pain-free for at least a week.

When training in the low-rep range or when you raise the amount of weight lifted by more than 5-10 pounds, you should always have a spotter nearby. In fact, it's smart to use a spotter every time you perform an exercise that could be dangerous if your muscles were to give out, such as the bench press or the barbell squat. If you are by yourself, avoid pushing yourself to failure while using free weights. If you want to go to failure and you're by yourself, use machines for your workout, which won't "pin" you or otherwise put you in danger if your muscles give out.

Other safety tips for working out include:
– Wear closed-toe shoes or sneakers, the more durable the better in case a weight gets dropped on your toes.
–Make sure that the area is clear when you are ready to start your set and that there is nothing that might startle you during your set.
–Make sure you have had enough food and drink so you don't feel faint during exercise. Sip water or a sports drink such as Gatorade during your workout.
–It is preferable to avoid exercising alone. If you must, tell someone when you're leaving and when you're expected back. Bring a cell phone with you.
–If you're going to exercise outside on the road, wear light clothing with reflective material.
–Use protective gear suited for your activity, such as a helmet for outdoor cycling.
–Make sure to use sunscreen if you're exercising outdoors.
–If you have asthma or sometimes suffer from exercise-induced asthma, have your inhaler with you at all times during your workouts.

Besides the safety precautions you need to take during workouts, there are safety issues surrounding supplement use. Be wary of pills advertised as "fat-burners" or "thermogenic formulas." Many of them contain large amounts of caffeine. While this shouldn't harm you any more than a large cup of coffee, if you're drinking coffee or cola *and* taking a couple of fat-burner pills per day, you're going to have way too much caffeine in your system. Avoid the thermogenics that contain ephedra or other herbal stimulants you're not familiar with. Ephedra has been banned from sale in the U.S. due to many complaints and even some deaths associated with the use of this substance, but I'm sure there are still some bottles kicking around.

If you're considering taking any of these fat burner formulas, you need to thoroughly research the substance or run the list of ingredients by a professional. Even then, know that you are playing Russian roulette by taking these supplements, because it's hard to say if they *really* contain what the label *says* they contain. Sometimes the supplement will contain less of the active ingredient than the label claims because the company is trying to increase it's profit margin, while other times a "mystery" ingredient has been added to increase the effectiveness of the supplement or to cut down on manufacturing costs by using a cheaper substitute (in this case you'll have no way of knowing potential side effects). Sometimes the company isn't necessarily trying to pull a fast one – it's just that it has poor quality control and every bottle ends up containing more or less of the active ingredient that's indicated on the label.

Even if your supplement is labeled accurately, some supplements can be harmful to certain individuals, particularly if you happen to be taking any medications that might interact with the active ingredient in the supplement.

All safety questions aside, do supplements really work? Do they do what they say they'll do? The average person is most interested in the various types of diet pills. There are three main categories of diet pills that "work" by different mechanisms. The first category is the thermogenic formulas. Most of the thermogenics do "work" to a point – they offer the dieter a slight advantage *as long as you're already running a calorie deficit.* In some cases they help you burn extra calories (they increase your metabolism), but the true figure for extra calories burned is almost always less than 100 calories per day, or about the equivalent of one slice of bread. At that rate, it would take over two months to lose one pound as a direct result of taking these supplements. Some of the thermogenics work by affecting what *type* of weight you lose – the better ones promote the loss of bodyfat and help spare muscle tissue. However, a good exercise program and diet plan will do that – and if you don't have the exercise and diet part down, the pills won't do a thing. To summarize, a thermogenic formula might promote fat loss to a slight degree, but most of the time the difference between using those formulas along with diet and exercise and diet and exercise alone is negligible. *The thermogenics won't do much of anything if your diet and exercise routine isn't top notch.* If you haven't been losing weight without the pills, these formulas won't save you, although using them *will* drain your bank account pretty quickly. Also, realize that your body will adapt to the presence of these supplements, meaning that any progress you make on them is likely to be short-lived since your body will be primed to gain the fat back once you go off them. And you *will* want to go off them, because you will stop seeing results after a little while and may even revert in progress since your body will usually downgrade its own systems in order to compensate for the presence of a foreign substance. Your body likes to maintain a state of homeostasis, and when you introduce a new substance into your system you are interfering with your body's natural functioning.

While the thermogenic formulas are designed to help elevate your metabolism, there are other diet pills that claim to work by blocking the absorption of fats or carbohydrates. We'll call this category of diet pills the "blockers." It's simple to explain the story on these things, because it's really a no-win situation – either the pills don't block enough calories to make a difference, or they do – but in that case you'll be on the toilet all day with diarrhea. You'll be passing some of the food through your system without it being digested properly, and even then the pills won't eliminate *all* the calories from the food. I don't believe anyone should use the "blockers" because there's no reason why you can't keep your energy balance at the right level for weight loss simply by eating the proper amount of food and exercising. And if you follow the 80/20 Rule with your diet, you will be able to go off your plan at times and still lose weight – without needing expensive pills that cause diarrhea and malnutrition (vitamins and minerals in your food get passed through your system as well if the pills "work" for you).

The third category of diet pills is the appetite suppressants. These actually might be the most effective of the three types of diet pills, simply because they make it easier to keep your calorie intake where it needs to be for weight loss. The different appetite suppressants work by a variety of mechanisms, but all are supposed to reduce your hunger and/or appetite. What was so great about ephedra (it's since been banned) is that it acts as a thermogenic *and* an appetite suppressant. However, better than 99 out of 100 people don't need an appetite suppressant to achieve long-term weight-loss – they simply need to learn how to make better food choices that help control hunger, appetite, and cravings. The only people who really have a use for appetite suppressants at times are pro-bodybuilders looking to drop into the low single digits in bodyfat percentage, and the morbidly obese whose lives are in danger from overeating. One of the problems with appetite suppressants is that they tend to work for only a few weeks before the effects begin to wear off, so they must be used judiciously. A behavior modification program must accompany the administration of appetite suppressants to justify their use.

Medications classified as appetite suppressants act upon the body's central nervous system, tricking the body into believing it's not hungry. The list of prescription appetite suppressants includes benzphetamine, diethylpropion, mazindol and phentermine (9). These medications generally come in the form of tablets or extended-release capsules. Appetite suppressants can be prescribed or purchased over-the-counter. Just like with the blockers, you'll tend to encounter the problem of using something that is too weak to have much of an effect, or else you'll find that it works *too* well. If your appetite suppressant is too powerful, you'll have trouble eating *enough* to prevent your metabolism from slowing down. The other problem with these pills is that they can work well at first, but you'll find that you enjoy the desired effects for just a short time, only to be left with the unpleasant side effects. Here is a short list of those side effects:

- increased heart rate
- increased blood pressure
- sweating
- constipation
- insomnia
- excessive thirst
- lightheadedness
- drowsiness

I have yet to work with a client who required an appetite suppressant to lose weight. Following a moderate-protein, moderate-fat, moderate-carb diet that includes plenty of dietary fiber, eating every 3 or 4 hours, and exercising works like a charm to manage your weight, with no side effects other than losing weight and looking great.

While the majority of people in the U.S. who want to change their appearance would like to lose bodyfat, others have the primary goal of building muscle and/or gaining weight. These folks are looking at a different category of supplements. Regular steroids, typically in the form of injectable testosterone, are illegal but still popular among bodybuilders. "Legal steroids," collectively known as "andro," are currently in vogue among bodybuilders and also among "regular" guys in the gym who want to make faster gains (you can get them right at your local GNC). In a nutshell, "andro" is a category of prohormones that aids in testosterone production. Most of them are a direct hormone precursor to testosterone (whereas illegal steroids *are* testosterone), which is why they are so effective but still able to avoid the legality issue, at least for the time being. Andros are just one chemical step away from testosterone, and the human body is able to convert this legal substance into a substance that would be illegal if it were injected directly. As you can imagine, increasing the amount of testosterone in the body in any way, shape or form results in bigger muscles for the person who's weight training. What you may not realize is that testosterone also makes it easier to be *both bigger and leaner* than would be possible drug-free.

Normally, there is a ceiling to how much muscle a "natural" (non-steroid using) person can gain before it's inevitable that they gain some fat along with it. Having higher testosterone levels changes all that. It literally allows the human body to defy the laws of nature. Having higher testosterone levels also defends against the tendency for the metabolism to crash in response to dieting. Artificial testosterone is the reason that elite bodybuilders can get both freakishly big and freakishly lean. They eat huge amounts of calories to gain weight, and because they're on steroids or andro, most of that added weight comes in the form of muscle. Then they go on a superstrict diet and shed the fat, without experiencing the drop in metabolism that one would expect on such a drastic diet, again due to the extra testosterone. It's a safe bet that the vast majority of bodybuilders, men and women alike, are literally "jacked up" on some form of testosterone, whether it be from andro or steroid use.

It's becoming more and more widespread for everyone from teenage boys to your average guy in the gym to experiment with andro. While this might seem like a magic way to gain muscle fast, andro has its dark side. There's no reason why you need to build more muscle than you can acquire naturally from working out hard and eating right. If you insist upon building more muscle or would like to use a supplement to maximize the effort you're making in the gym, there are other supplements that can help you gain muscle and carry nowhere near the risks that come with taking andro. The most proven of this group is creatine, and it is virtually free of side effects, yet effective for most people. In my opinion, there is no reason why anyone should take andro. Apparently others agree – the FDA is in the process of banning the sale of prohormones because it's becoming apparent that they lead to many of the same problems we see with illegal steroid use. Side effects of andro include (10):

For both men and women:
- kidney and liver damage
- acne problems and oily skin
- lowered HDL cholesterol (the good kind)
- weakening of the bones, leading to full-blown osteoporosis

For men:
- premature baldness
- enlarged prostates, reduced sperm production, and increased aggression
- shrinkage of testicles, infertility, loss of libido, and impotence

For women:
- disruption of menstrual cycles
- deepened voice and increased facial hair
- enlargement of the clitoris

Better safe than sorry assignment

1. If you develop pain anywhere in the body, don't ignore it. Try to discover the root of the problem before things get worse. If it doesn't go away on it's own after a day or two, you'll need to rest the injured area for at least a few days to let yourself heal, and you may have to make a change in your workout routine. A visit to an orthopedic doctor might be in order.

2. Get in the habit of double-checking your surroundings to be sure that you're safe during your workouts. Always let someone know you are leaving to exercise if you plan to exercise alone. Also, make sure you've taken care of your physical needs, meaning that you've had enough food and drink and enough rest/sleep. Make sure you're wearing the appropriate clothing and gear for your activity and the weather.

3. Never take a supplement without researching it thoroughly, and take all warning labels seriously. *Never* administer more than the dose indicated on the label without consulting a professional. If you are currently taking any medications, including over-the-counter and herbal treatments, be sure to talk to a professional before you take any supplement.

Strategy 21: 48-hour rule – Leave that muscle alone!

How rest allows you to progress even faster

Muscles need approximately 48 hours to recover after a resistance-training workout. The reason is that weight training or challenging bodyweight exercises cause small tears in your muscle fibers, particularly when you reach muscular fatigue by 12 reps. During the 24-48 hours following your training session, the protein available in your body from food you've had that day (and sometimes from your body's own muscle tissue, since your body is capable of burning muscle as a fuel source) will be put to work repairing the damaged muscle fibers. The end result is that you build stronger, harder muscles when you train them the right way and allow enough time for recovery.

You can, however, work other muscles in your body the very next day without interfering with this recovery process. For instance, if you work your chest by doing push-ups and the bench press, the next day you could work your legs by doing squats and lunges. There's no need to skip a day in between if you'll be hitting different muscles.

Just remember that you still need to keep total workout volume in check within your workout week. In other words, it's no problem to lift weights two days in a row as long as you don't hit the same area, but you still need to take a break from lifting altogether some days. You need enough rest in your schedule to allow your system to recover from the generalized stress that working out places on your body. Your central nervous system and immune system perceive working out in any way, shape, or form as a stress on your entire body, which means even if you keep changing the area of your body you work, you still need to rest from *all* activity at times.

For most people, at least one full day per week with no formal workout is in order (walking isn't included in that recommendation – it's fine to walk on a daily basis). Beginners need to build up the capacity of their central nervous system to handle stress, and therefore are advised to perform resistance-training no more than every other day. A full body resistance-training program performed three times per week is ideal for beginners. Moderate to vigorous cardio can also be performed three days per week, either on the same day or on alternate days from the resistance training. Your system will eventually adapt to a greater workload if you'd like to do more, as long as you don't overburden it too much in the beginning.

Once you've adapted to the stress that weight training places on your body, you will be prepared to move into a split routine if you wish. A split routine is one in which you work only some of your muscle groups on a given day – for example, day 1 might be upper body and day 2 might be lower body. If your primary goal is weight loss, it's not necessary or even desirable in most cases to use split routines, but they *can* be used as part of a weight loss program if you're planning to lift nearly every day. For weight loss, you'll get the best results if you exercise all the muscles in your body 2-3 times a week. That means, unless you're planning to lift 4-6 times per week (with each workout only hitting half the muscles in the body), split routines are not for you. To build muscle as a natural lifter, the recommendation is the same: Your best bet is to exercise all the muscles in your body 2-3 times a week. You could accomplish this with full-body workouts or with a split routine.

Keep in mind that your central nervous system can be stressed from other activities besides exercise. That's one reason why your body won't respond as well to exercise if you're sleep-deprived, calorie-deprived, or under mental or emotional strain. All these stressors will tax you, leaving less energy for your workouts and your recovery from those workouts. And, *recovery* is actually how you get stronger and improve your body composition. Too much stress is harmful to your figure and your health. For best results, apply a stress to your body with the workouts and then rest to allow your body to respond. The adaptation is what you're after – the workouts are just a means to get there. That's why you need to rest if you want to get the full benefit from working out.

Do you remember what I said about stress levels, the hormone cortisol, and abdominal fat? Your body will flat-out refuse to shed the last bit of excess bodyfat if you're overworking yourself. Too much exercise with too little rest has the same effect on your body and your metabolism as cutting calories too hard — your body will respond by dropping muscle and hoarding fat. You've got to strike a balance between training and rest in order to look your best. If you turn to the tables in Reference D you'll see that inadequate rest and high stress levels take away points from your "fitness score" and will prevent you from getting into the best of shape.

48 hour rule – Leave that muscle alone! assignment

1. Make sure your program includes the appropriate amount of rest for each muscle group, as well as enough rest overall. If you don't have any weeklong vacations or business trips coming up during which you won't be able to or won't want to work out, be sure to plan rest periods into your workout schedule. In general, resistance training 3-5 days per week for 45-60 minutes at a time and cardio for about the same is the most you can do per week on a regular basis (even as an advanced exerciser) without putting yourself on the fast track to burnout. Also, avoid working the same muscle group more than three times per week. If you're not sure how much work is best for you, or how you should split your routine, have a trainer look at your program, or check out those resources in Reference E for some sample routines.

Strategy 22: The stronger, the better

How to use strength and performance as a results indicator

There are two ways that your body can get stronger. The first is by building more muscle, which means increasing the size of the muscle fibers. The second is by improving the conditioning of the neurological pathways to your muscles. This gives you better control of the muscle you already have. No matter which way you get stronger, it's always a good sign when your strength increases. Why?

1. An increase in strength means that you have become more fit, which is good for your health and also improves your appearance.
2. If the calories you eat are being burned off during training and in the process of building and repairing muscle, they won't be stored as fat and your body is more likely to burn bodyfat for energy.
3. Well-developed muscle tissue is what gives your body a toned look, and when your strength goes up your body will look and feel firmer.
4. As your strength goes up, you will be able to work out harder, which leads to an increase in lean body mass and/or a decrease in fat mass over time. This increases your metabolism and makes it easier to reach or maintain a healthy bodyweight.

Increases in strength are a good indication that you're on the right track to having the body you've always wanted. Improving your fitness automatically means improving your looks, your energy level, and your health. You can never go wrong by improving your fitness and getting stronger.

Beginners can usually lose fat and gain muscle at the same time when they begin a resistance-training program. However, after your first month or two of consistent training, it becomes virtually impossible to gain significant amounts of muscle and lose significant amounts of fat at the same time. If you are restricting calories and/or carbohydrates or losing weight for some other reason, you will be fortunate to maintain your strength, let alone increase it. You won't gain much, if any strength while losing weight unless you are a beginner or are returning from a long hiatus from working out. This phenomenon is called "beginner gains" because that's the only time you can expect to build significant amounts of muscle and gain strength while losing bodyfat at the same time.

In general, after the beginner phase you will see the quickest success with your physique goals when you focus on either muscle building (hopefully while keeping fat gain to a minimum) or fat loss (hopefully while keeping muscle loss to a minimum). The reason is that the hormonal milieu when you're running the calorie deficit that's required for fat loss is completely different from the hormonal picture when you're in the calorie surplus that's necessary to build muscle.

Advanced exercisers who are serious about building or maintaining muscle and also losing fat will typically alternate periods of gaining muscle and losing fat, with a complete cycle taking as little as one week or as long as six months to complete. During each cycle, the person spends some time running a calorie deficit and some time in a calorie surplus. This is the most efficient way to change your body composition because the body is either anabolic (building tissue) or catabolic (burning tissue) at any given time. To make a significant change in the amount of muscle or fat on your body, you must remain in either the anabolic or the catabolic phase for a period of time (at least three days, but typically a couple of weeks to see a significant change). Once in a while you'll find people who can gain muscle and lose fat at the same time, but that's only because they're genetically lean and have a low set point for bodyfat. If you're like the majority of people, you *will* have to jump through hoops if you want to be "ripped" (6-pack abs and chiseled arms and legs). The people that go this route are your athletes, models, bodybuilders, and figure competitors, and even those who are just vain and/or like to work out. The truth is that most people that are successful in getting super-lean have a genetic predisposition to be lean anyway, and they couple that predisposition with hard work and discipline to get their stellar results. That means your "average joe" who works just as hard and diets just as strictly will never look as good as the person with better genetics for being lean. Keep in mind, too, that athletes, models, and figure/bodybuilding competitors usually have an "off" season during which they relax their regimen and allow themselves to get a little out-of-shape (which, to the rest of us, still seems "in shape!")

Unless you have lofty fitness goals, you won't need to train for hours or follow a cyclic dieting plan to get in shape. The average person just looking to get in better shape won't need to get that fancy or particular with diet and training. Most of my clients aren't involved in the advanced methods or simply the annoying ones like counting calories and the like – it's not necessary to go to those lengths just to look healthy and trim and be in good shape. If you want to look and feel better and be healthier, being relatively consistent with exercise and proper nutrition over time should get you to where you want to be. Most people will be able to reach a healthy weight and bodyfat percentage following a basic approach, which includes performing cardio and weights 2-3 times a week and following a good diet most of the time.

The stronger, the better assignment

1. As you go through your workouts, keep track of your weight and reps for each exercise and strive for consistent increases in strength. Try increasing the amount of weight you use for an exercise once you are able to perform 15 reps with good form. During the first six months of a program, adding anything from 2.5 to 25 pounds per month to a lift is good progress (the range is given to accommodate the different types of exercises and the differences in strength between males and females). Keep in mind that you might not be able to increase the amount of weight you lift if you are losing bodyweight. You still should do your best to at least maintain your lifts, though. If you manage to maintain your lifts while losing bodyweight, your strength-to-weight ratio will actually go up. For instance, consider a 140-pound woman who squats 100 pounds for eight reps. If she loses 10 pounds but still can squat 100 pounds for eight reps, her strength-to-weight ratio for the squat goes from 100/140 (0.71) to 100/130 (0.77). On the other hand, if she gains 10 pounds (putting her at 150) but can't lift any more than she did when she weighed 140, she's actually getting weaker according to her strength-to-weight ratio of 100/150 (0.67).

This goes to show that strength isn't as straightforward as the number of pounds a person can lift. Besides looking at the strength-to-weight ratio, there are other instances where you can demonstrate an increase in strength without actually increasing the number of pounds you use for an exercise. If you improve your form on an exercise and still lift the same weight for the same number of reps, the fact that you are able to use more control and isolate the muscles you're supposed to be working demonstrates that you are getting stronger and performing better.

When comparing strength, you also have to keep the implications of training specificity in mind. Let's look at the case where one person performs cardio and weights and the other just trains with weights. Even if both spend the same amount of time weightlifting, the person who only does weights will get stronger faster. The same holds true for the person who just does cardio – he will be able to go faster for longer during cardio than the person who does both weighs and cardio. This is because muscles develop in accordance with the stimulus you provide through your training. If you only do one type of activity, your muscles will "specialize" and develop only with the purpose of performing that activity better. On the other hand, if you do two different activities using the same muscle, your muscle will "compromise" and develop in a manner to accommodate both activities.

A person who does cardio and weights uses his legs for both activities, which means that the legs will be forced to develop endurance and strength. The person who only lifts weights will specialize his legs for strength and will develop stronger legs because the muscles won't have to dedicate any muscle fibers to increasing endurance capacity. That doesn't mean it's recommended to stick to just one type of exercise, though! The person who does a variety of workouts incorporating cardio and weights as well as explosive/athletic training will be the "fittest" of them all and will have much better endurance and power and usually a lower bodyfat percentage than the person who only does one of the three types of workouts. You just need to understand that you're comparing apples and oranges when you compare yourself to someone in one particular activity where he happens to be a "specialist" if you do a variety of activities.

If your main goal is weight loss or having a toned body, you should definitely incorporate all types of training in your routine. A truly fit person excels in many areas of fitness, but will never become the world champion in any of them because he hasn't specialized his muscles to any one activity.

Another neat thing to know about muscles is that they are capable of adapting to any type of training. Even if you think you weren't "built" to be a runner or a powerlifter, if you keep training for that activity your body will start adapting and your physique will begin approaching the ideal musculature for that sport. This won't be a permanent change, though – if you stop practicing one sport and start another, your muscles will begin adapting for the new activity. While the ability to adapt means that you have more options for activities you can do, it also explains why you'll fall out of shape pretty quickly if you don't do anything at all. If you become a couch potato, your muscles will "adapt" to doing nothing!

Think about the difference in appearance between a marathon runner and a sprinter, or a bodybuilder and a powerlifter. Sure, some of the differences are due to genetics, but those athletes have all trained themselves in a specific way for their particular sport. Depending on which type of training you choose, you can develop the ability to do virtually any activity you desire, including things such as running long distances, heavy weightlifting, and the high jump. That doesn't mean you'll do all of them very *well* if you're not a natural, but you can still develop skill and make great progress.

As you develop skills and abilities for a particular sport or type of training, your performance typically changes at a faster rate than your physique. In other words, if you start running long distances and you have a bulky build (not a lean and streamlined one like good long-distance runners typically have) you will become a better runner fairly quickly even if your body doesn't visibly change much. Everyone has a genetic predisposition toward a certain body type, and you can only alter it so much. That's why it isn't always the best idea to simply start training like someone who has a body that you admire. The same exercises will produce different results for different bodies. Many of the best training protocols for changing your physique are actually quite counterintuitive. You don't want to copy someone else's program simply because they have the look you want. They probably look that way due to genetics more than anything else, and in some cases look the way they do *in spite of* how they train! I've seen people with great muscle development who train in a way that makes very little sense physiologically, but they look great anyway because it's in their genetics. Don't get discouraged, though – I've also seen people with average genetics who developed their bodies through the proper diet and training and look phenomenal. Two people can train exactly the same way and have drastically different results because they have different genetics, different body types, and different starting points. You need to find the best workout for you and follow the recommendations as closely as you can.

To bring this concept home, think about what happens when you go into a hair salon asking for a particular haircut. Let's suppose that you show the stylist a picture of a haircut you like and ask if he can give you that cut. Hopefully your hair type is conducive to your request. If it's not and the stylist agrees to try the cut anyway, chances are the cut is not going to come out like you hoped.

Let's assume that the cut is appropriate for your hair type and it comes out pretty close to the picture you brought in. Still, due to differences in facial structure, facial features, and coloring, the cut will never look quite the same as it does in the picture. This goes to show that there's only so much you can do given the limitations of genetics. Getting back to bodies, though, there's still no reason why anyone should carry excess bodyfat and too little muscle, no matter what his body type. Everyone can make improvements on what he has and make the most of the genetic hand he's been dealt. Read through Reference D to understand your body type and to get an idea which training modalities will suit you best.

Strategy 23: Just right

Choosing the right resistance

Generally, you should choose the heaviest weight you can handle with correct form for your resistance training. If you are an intermediate or advanced exerciser, you will want to have heavy low-rep days (sets to muscular failure at 3-6 reps) mixed in with medium-weight, medium-rep days and light, high-rep days (sets to muscular failure at 7-12 or 12-15 reps, respectively) in order to progress at the fastest pace with minimal risk of injury. Heavy training isn't only for powerlifters or bodybuilders – anyone who wants to get stronger and have a higher metabolism should use heavy low-rep training at times.

Sometimes it makes sense to train with a weight that you're not even capable of lifting by yourself. This amount of weight is good for "negatives," an advanced technique where the lifter gets help lifting the weight from a spotter, but lowers it slowly and under control with no assistance. Everyone is stronger on the "lowering" portion of a rep, and training negatives takes advantage of this phenomenon, allowing you to apply even more tension to the muscle. "Negatives," then, are one tool you have for increasing the resistance used while exercising. Training with negatives is a great way to increase strength and break through a fitness plateau.

Another related technique is forced reps. For forced reps, you keep pushing out more reps with a light spot after you can't do any more on your own. You continue to lower the weight on your own during forced reps, only allowing your spotter to assist you in lifting the weight. Forced reps, like negatives, take advantage of the fact that you're stronger lowering a weight than you are lifting it. Forced reps also allow you to recruit more muscle fibers than you would if you stopped after hitting muscular failure initially. Beginners shouldn't attempt advanced heavy low-rep sets, negatives, or forced reps until they've been training for at least two months. Always have a spotter on hand when you're working with heavy low-rep sets or using intensity techniques such as negatives and forced reps.

Now let's switch gears and talk about the opposite extreme in weightlifting: Many people are guilty of choosing a weight that is too light to stimulate their muscle tissue to adapt. Using a weight that you can lift for more than 15 reps at a time doesn't cause your body to change much, if at all. This type of light resistance work doesn't burn enough calories to take the place of cardio, yet the weights aren't heavy enough to force your muscles to adapt.

To understand why, you must realize that your body uses two separate systems during activity: The aerobic system and the anaerobic system. High-rep weight training isn't the most effective way to exercise either system. Technically, a set consisting of more than 15 reps or that takes over 60-90 seconds to complete is exercising the *aerobic system* in spite of the fact that you're lifting weights. The two systems don't operate on a continuum, so you can't get "the best of both worlds" by trying to do something in between. You are much better off doing a steady cardiovascular exercise like running to exercise your aerobic system and rounding out your program with heavier weight-training sessions to exercise your anaerobic system. Lifting weights for 15+ reps at a time builds muscular endurance, but won't improve your strength, build muscle, or result in fat loss nearly to the degree that a program including regular cardio and heavier weights will.

Many of the problems people have with exercising most effectively can be traced to gender differences. Women have a tendency to lift weights that are too light to change their bodies or stimulate their metabolism much, whereas men have a tendency to lift heavier weights than they are capable of handling with correct form, which compromises their results and puts them at risk for injury.

One reason women sometimes fail to push themselves on the weights is that many have fallen pray to the myth that lifting heavy weights makes you big and bulky. If women had as much testosterone as men, then sure, this *could* happen. The reality is that it's extremely rare to find a woman who has high enough testosterone levels that she *might* be able to build a physique similar to a "natural" male (a weightlifter not on steroids), and even then, *the only way people can gain weight is if they eat more calories than they burn.* Lifting heavy weights won't make you gain one ounce unless you're eating above-maintenance calories. It's true that some people experience an increase in appetite when they lift heavy weights, but if you follow a healthy diet you'll be able to eat plenty of food without gaining weight, and should be able to lose weight if you need to as long as you're watching your calories and doing cardio. Also, resistance training using heavy weights burns lots of calories, and therefore helps with weight loss in that sense.

If all these things I'm saying are true, you might be wondering how female bodybuilders get all that muscle. Most, if not all, of the women you've seen in bodybuilding are using andro or steroids. They're also consuming a very high-calorie diet during their bulking phases to put on all that muscle mass. They look the way they do as a result of the drugs and muscle-building supplements they use coupled with a very-high-calorie diet for at least part of the year. I know people who lift weights just as heavy as the female bodybuilders, and because they aren't eating as much or taking steroids they don't have very big muscles in spite of how much weight they lift. It's simply not in the female genotype to have big muscles, no matter what type of exercise they do. If a woman's arm or leg looks too big, at least 99 times out of 100 it's due to a layer of fat over the muscles. Women who feel "too big" need to target that bodyfat through diet and exercise – they don't need to reduce the size of their muscles. You're bound to lose some muscle when you're dieting anyway, and you want to spare as much as possible because muscle is what helps keep your body firm and your metabolism high. Maybe you *are* bigger-boned and have larger muscles than some of your petite friends, but you're shooting yourself in the foot if you *try* to lose muscle. You'll be facing a lifetime of starving yourself and yo-yo dieting if you try to make your body into something it's not. If you weren't born to be a waif, you can save yourself a lot of grief by giving up the idea of trying to look like one. You'll look and feel *your* best when you eat properly, perform resistance training, and reduce your bodyfat levels with a combination of weights, cardio, and diet. I know this might not be what you want to hear, but it's the truth.

Even after they've pushed the fear of developing large muscles aside, women usually need to be encouraged to do more on the weights because they are generally less aggressive in the gym than men. This is, again, due mainly to differences in testosterone levels. Testosterone is the reason guys are able to lift more than gals, even when comparing a man and women who are the same height and who both carry the same amount of muscle on their body. Of course, men usually outweigh women in the muscle department, so most men have a double advantage that allows them to lift so much more than women, assuming that genetic potential has been reached. In summary, it's true that guys usually have more muscle weight on their bodies than women, but they also can lift more pound-for-pound.

It's certainly possible to find a fit woman who can outlift an out-of-shape man, but a fit man always outlifts a fit woman. All the testosterone that makes men so physically strong also fosters a tendency to act aggressively. Men are much more likely than women to be guilty of "throwing the weight around" meaning to use momentum and lift too fast, and are more likely to get hurt because they were trying to lift too much. They are also more likely to try to "work through" an injury when they're hurting, which is almost always counterproductive to long-term progress. On the other hand, aggressiveness in the gym can also be an asset. Men usually push themselves quite a bit during their workouts, and as long as it's done within reason, this will accelerate their progress.

Most men don't gravitate to cardio like females tend to, and this is due in part to hormonal differences. Men prefer short but intense bursts of exertion as a general rule. This makes sense because testosterone gives men the capacity to exert at a higher level during exercise. Women generally prefer lower levels of exertion but will happily work for longer periods at a time. This means they tend to prefer long, light sets during resistance training and they usually don't mind moderate-pace cardio.

Besides the hormonal differences, there's another issue affecting exercise preferences between men and women – it has to do with fuel usage during exercise. Everyone uses carbs to fuel resistance training. When it comes to cardio, however, men burn carbs preferentially over fat for fuel, whereas females burn fat more readily (This is ironic because women carry more bodyfat than men as a general rule and have a harder time mobilizing stubborn fat. This paradox is something that still befuddles top exercise physiologists).

Remember, carbs are an anaerobic, or high-exertion fuel. Any high-intensity or high-exertion exercise such as heavy resistance training, sprints, or explosive movements such as those made while playing sports is going to rely strictly on carbs for fuel. That's why you'll see men willing to run around to play pick-up basketball, but it can be like pulling teeth to get them on the treadmill for a 45-minute jog. Men tend to use carbs for both aerobic and anaerobic activities, which means that they "run out" of carbs faster than women. To make matters worse, men have a harder time using fat for fuel even once their carb stores are depleted, and therefore generally struggle to do long sessions of cardio unless they train consistently for it. Stop-and-start activities use strictly carbs for fuel, which is one of the reasons why men tend to prefer and perform better at them.

Women, on the other hand, burn fat just fine during cardio. Fat is a longer-lasting fuel and purely an aerobic fuel. When you use fat for fuel, you don't experience the burning sensation in the muscles that you get when you use carbs for fuel (This burning sensation is due to lactic acid buildup, a byproduct of carbohydrate metabolism). Since they are less likely to experience that burning sensation because they're using fat for fuel, women tend to prefer aerobics and usually would rather do a long set of 15+ reps with a lighter weight than a shorter set of 6-8 reps with heavier weight (remember, I said that a long set like this becomes aerobic and therefore can be fueled partially with fat). Men have no choice but to tolerate the lactic acid burn since they don't burn fat as readily, but the burn also makes it harder for them to continue for long periods of time doing aerobics or high-rep sets. Of course, all of these observations are general *tendencies* and do not apply to everyone. Moreover, gravitating toward one activity or another does *not* mean that men and women should work out much differently.

It's true that men's and women's bodies are a bit different structurally, which does affect the way the muscles work to a slight degree. The biggest difference, though, isn't so much the structural variation between men and women but rather the hormonal milieu that serves as a backdrop for all the processes that take place in the body.

In spite of that, however, men and women have the same muscle groups to exercise, which means that their lifting regimens should be roughly the same. Both may need cardio, depending on how their diet is and what their goals are. Women usually need more cardio than men to get lean because they have a smaller body size and carry less muscle mass, which means they burn fewer calories. The extra calories burned through cardio can be a big help for a woman to create a sufficient calorie deficit to lose weight. Women also have more of the "stubborn fat" that is almost impossible to mobilize without cardio.

Unfortunately, this extra need for cardio doesn't preclude women from needing as much resistance training as guys if they want to get really lean. Ladies, it doesn't seem fair now, does it? The reality is that women have to fight harder against nature if they want to have an athletic body because women are *programmed* to carry more bodyfat than men. This extra bodyfat is necessary for a woman to be ready to nourish a fetus if she were to get pregnant.

What ends up happening when picking apart people's exercise routines is that I usually need to push guys to get all their cardio done, whereas women usually need to be pushed to exert more on the weights. It's important for everyone to focus on the areas they tend to avoid or shortchange. In the end, the ideal workout program for a woman isn't much different from the ideal workout program for a man. There will be a few differences, however. Females usually lift quite a bit less weight, although the weight they choose should still be very challenging for them. Most males won't need quite as much cardio. Those two issues aside, men and women should work out the same way, using the same lifts and performing the same types of cardio. If you take a workout plan that includes weights and cardio and give it to a male and a female, instructing both individuals to lift the most they can and to be consistent with their cardio, the end result will be a sexy, shapely figure for the woman and a "ripped," muscular body for the man.

Just right assignment

1.   Make sure you are using the appropriate weight for each exercise and the appropriate degree of difficulty with your bodyweight exercises. Remember to periodically assess whether the resistance you're using should be changed, and try experimenting with heavier weights and tougher bodyweight exercises as an intermediate or advanced lifter. If you're interested in varying your resistance training in a systematic fashion, you can learn more about training cycles in the upcoming Strategies as well as in Reference C under the subheading, "Progressive Resistance Cycle Training." The websites listed in Reference E can provide additional ideas for your workouts.

Strategy 24: Racking up those miles

How cardiovascular work fits into the picture

Cardiovascular exercise is the best thing you can do for heart-health, and it's also a great weight-loss tool. Although I believe that resistance training is superior to cardiovascular training for long-term weight maintenance and overall health, I am a firm believer in including cardio as part of anyone's exercise routine. Most people will be see far superior results if they do both cardio and weights.

The reason I place resistance training above cardio in its importance for fitness is that you can get some of the same benefits of cardio through resistance training (such as elevating your heart rate and burning calories). You also can get some of the effects of cardio during everyday life (such as having a moderate activity level and burning extra calories). You don't get *any* of the benefits of resistance training as a result of doing cardio, however. There is simply no substitute for resistance training, and the benefits are far too numerous to pass up.

Besides the increase in metabolism and the improvement in glucose metabolism (which leads to a reduced risk of heart disease and diabetes, a decrease in bodyfat, and increased energy level) you will have stronger bones and maintain your youthfulness and vigor much longer when you do resistance training. Did you know that weight training has a greater effect on improving bone-density than taking calcium supplements (11)? Both are important, of course, but the calcium supplements won't do much if your bones aren't placed under physical stress on a regular basis. Stress on the bones (which you get during resistance training) is the prerequisite that stimulates your bones to take up calcium. You have to place *all* the bones in your body under tension in order to develop a strong skeletal system. High-impact cardiovascular exercise will stimulate the bones in the lower body, but won't do anything for the bones in the upper body. And if your cardio is low-impact (such as cycling, swimming, or walking) it won't do a thing for your bone strength. A full-body resistance-training program is an efficient way to cover all bases for your bone strength.

How many elderly people do you know whose health started deteriorating after they fell and broke a wrist or hip? If you're like me, you know quite a few. If these people had maintained a resistance training routine most of their life, they wouldn't be as susceptible to broken bones and probably could have preserved their quality of life for at least a few more years. In fact, they might not have fallen at all if they were stronger and had better balance, both of which are developed through a well-designed exercise routine.

Although resistance training is important in so many ways, a formal cardio workout is extremely beneficial not only for weight loss but also for improving endurance, heart health, and energy level, and you cannot ignore cardio if your goal is to be fit and healthy.

If you're just starting out, begin training your cardiovascular system by walking or using a stationary bike for 10-20 minutes, two days per week. Work up to spending 30 minutes, 2-3 times a week on cardio. That is all the cardio you need if your goal is simply to maintain heart health.

If your goal is accelerated fat loss or improved stamina, you'll need to increase your workout time to 30 minutes a session. Furthermore, you'll need to bump up the intensity once you are able to complete 30 minutes of easy to moderate-pace cardio. There are a number of ways to increase intensity. You can go faster during your cardio or go for longer, or you can increase the resistance you're working against. If you walk for your workout, increasing your intensity could mean increasing your speed or duration, or adding hills to your course.

In most cases, at the intermediate and advanced level you can train cardio for 30-60 minutes per day, 4-5 days per week without overburdening your system. If you are doing a high-intensity activity such as sprints or uphill running, 15-30 minutes is a more appropriate amount. Anything from 2-6 days of cardio per week can result in a high fitness level and accelerated fat loss, depending on the person and the activity. For most people, 3-5 days a week is ideal.

I would rather see someone work harder during three sessions a week than take it easier but do six. When your intensity is higher you'll experience greater adaptation from the exercise, which will improve your metabolism and your body composition. You'll also have more time off for recovery when you do fewer sessions, which is important in order to get the full benefit from your exercise program. You'll need to find the combination that works best for you, keeping in mind what is ideal physiologically as well as what works best for you psychologically. You'll also need to take into consideration how much time and effort you're willing to spend. Through trial and error you'll discover your ideal combination of hard and easy sessions. Following the advice of a trainer should help cut down on the amount of time you spend experimenting.

I know that less time can mean more result with cardio, and there are three main reasons why. The first is that appetite tends to increase when you're doing a good deal of cardiovascular work, especially after you hit a certain threshold (this threshold typically lies somewhere around 45-60 minutes per session, 5 days per week). What does this mean for your exercise program and your weight-loss goals? If you stick to 30-45 minutes of cardio, your appetite probably won't change much even though you will experience fat loss as long as you're in a calorie deficit. If you do more than 45-60 minutes, however, you might end up getting hungry enough that you overeat and compensate for all the exercise with a higher food intake, effectively negating those calories you burned. And if you fail to maintain a calorie deficit, no amount of cardio will result in fat loss.

Another reason less is sometimes more with cardio is that people tend to work harder (increase their exercise intensity) when they know they don't have to work for as long or as often. There are physical and psychological explanations for this phenomenon. Mentally you'll have better focus when you don't train as often, and physically you'll be fresher and will be able to offer up more intensity when it comes time for your sessions. If you work hard enough on your cardio, even if your workout is short, you will experience a post-exercise calorie burn in addition to the calories burned during the actual workout. This is why you don't get quite the same result by going slower and increasing the amount of time you exercise to try to make up for it. For example, if a person walks for 60 minutes at a speed of 4 m.p.h., he covers 4 miles and will burn about the same number of calories during his session as the person who jogs 4 miles at 8 m.p.h. (which would only take 30 minutes). Both covered 4 miles, although the walker took longer to do it. The calorie burn from walking or running is very similar on a per-mile basis. That is, covering one mile burns pretty close to the same number of calories whether you walk or run.

However, the difference comes when you look at the post-exercise calorie burn. The harder you push yourself beyond your comfort zone, the more calories you'll burn during the next 24 hours as your system adapts and recovers. The variables that are important when looking at total calorie burn as a result of exercise are distance, speed, incline or resistance, and effort. Distance has the greatest effect on the number of calories burned *during* the session, while speed, incline, and resistance are the variables that can increase the *post-exercise calorie burn*.

In general, shorter-duration but harder cardio (meaning you cover as much distance as possible in the least amount of time) is more effective for fat loss, especially for intermediate and advanced exercisers.

Beginners shouldn't try for speed yet – they need to ease themselves into a cardio routine to allow for cardiovascular adaptation to take place. Keeping an easy pace as a beginner will enable your cardiovascular system to adapt more efficiently. If you push too hard, your anaerobic system is apt to take over and your endurance won't improve as much. Getting your anaerobic system involved during "cardio" is actually a good technique to use at times as part of a fat-loss program, but if you're a beginner your first priority should be to train your cardio, or aerobic, system to become more efficient so that you will develop the capacity to burn a greater number of calories during your cardio sessions. Besides, the additional activity alone, no matter how "easy," does wonders for beginners. It's actually dangerous for beginners to try for a high level of exertion right away – their heart won't be equipped to handle it yet.

A third reason less can mean more with cardio is that your body always finds a way to adapt to the workload you do, and progress is apt to stall after you've been doing the same thing for a couple of months. If you are already doing, say, 10 hours of cardio a week, where are you supposed to go from there? At that rate, you can't keep adding more workout time to your schedule without suffering from a bad case of overtraining. Even if you decide to decrease your total workout time but increase your exercise intensity to make up for it, after spending so much time working out your body probably will have downgraded its basal metabolic rate because it felt threatened by all the energy you had been expending. It takes awhile for your body to "bounce back" again after you've abused it, so you'll find that you'll gain weight easily upon reducing your activity time when you've been doing a high volume of exercise.

It turns out that 3-5 sessions of cardio a week boosts the metabolism, but more than that starts to reverse the effects. If you burn *too many* calories through activity, your body will simply lower its basal metabolic rate, or BMR, to "save" calories. BMR refers to the number calories you burn per day before any activity, including the activities of daily living, is taken into account. Your body can lower its rate of calorie-burning by a number of mechanisms. One of those mechanisms is lowering the body temperature to conserve heat (which saves calories). Another way your body can lower its BMR is to reduce your energy level, which will limit your movement during daily life and will limit your energy expenditure during exercise, again resulting in calories saved.

Due to these reasons, six or more sessions of cardio per week should only be used for a specific purpose such as leaning out before an upcoming bodybuilding contest or improving performance before a race, and even then should only be used for short periods of time. Your body will tolerate that amount of stress for just a few weeks before it will downgrade your metabolism, which will halt any additional progress you would have made from training that frequently. The only exceptions where someone might be able to handle that much activity are when a person is extremely gifted genetically or when a person is taking hormones and/or drugs that keep the metabolism up (to counteract the drop that occurs with too much activity). You can always add more cardio if needed for some reason, so start out with 3-4 sessions a week even if you're eager to try more. Also, keep in mind that, if you're not losing bodyfat at an acceptable rate, changing your diet is probably going to make a bigger difference than adding a couple more cardio sessions.

If your goal is fat loss, avoid doing cardio right before your resistance training. Assuming you're also doing a resistance training program, you have three options for the best time to do cardio:

1. On the days you don't do resistance training.
2. On the same day but at a different time (meaning to leave at least three hours in between cardio and resistance training)
3. Immediately following your resistance training.

The only combination you should generally avoid is cardio followed immediately by resistance training. The reason has to do with fuel usage during exercise. I'll give you an overview on fuel usage so that the upcoming explanation will make sense.

Resistance training requires glucose for fuel (it's an anaerobic, or non-oxygen using, activity). Cardio, on the other hand, can be fueled by glucose or fat, depending on which is most readily available. Glucose molecules and fat molecules can be found circulating in the bloodstream almost all the time, assuming that you've had something to eat in the past 24 hours. Bodyfat can be mobilized into fat molecules and burned off for an additional source of fuel (By the way, this process can happen at any time during the day or night – burning bodyfat for fuel is not reserved for when you're exercising. Sitting, resting, and sleeping are technically all "aerobic" activities because they can rely on fat for fuel). Muscle tissue can be broken down to provide glucose, but this will only happen if your calorie deficit is too large (Hint – you don't want this to happen!).

If you have carbs and/or fat available in your bloodstream, your body will tend to fuel your cardio (and your daily living) with that nutrition first until that fuel source runs out. At that point, your body will start using bodyfat for fuel. The easiest thing for your body to do is burn carbs for fuel, so that's what it will do if there are any carbs available. Once you've used up most of your carb stores, fat-burning starts to pick up (this is one of the facts that the low-carb craze is based on). What you have to realize, however, is that carbs themselves aren't really the problem when someone struggles to lose bodyfat. It really doesn't matter whether you burn carbs or fat for fuel – the total number of calories burned, no matter what their source, is really what's important because, at the end of the day, weight loss will *always* be dictated by the magnitude of your calorie deficit. To lose weight, you'll need to burn more calories than you consume. So, it really doesn't matter what you use as fuel during daily activities and exercise, as long as your body doesn't have to resort to breaking down muscle for fuel. And that will only happen if you don't have enough fuel in your bloodstream to use.

It is true that some people lose more weight on low-fat diets and some lose more weight on low-carb diets. The primary reason is that some people maintain a calorie deficit more easily when they follow a low-fat diet, while others maintain a calorie deficit more easily when they follow a low-carb diet. This is partly due to variations in the way different people's bodies metabolize fat and carbs (some people handle a higher-carb diet better than others), but it's mainly due to plain-old appetite control. Whichever diet helps you control appetite and total calorie intake better will result in more weight loss for *you*. Good arguments can be made for low-carb and low-fat, but then again moderate-everything can work too. The only thing that *doesn't* work is high-calories all around, and that tends to happen when you take regular or oversized portion of high-fat and high-carb foods.

To prevent muscle breakdown during exercise, there are two things you need to avoid: Don't do cardio before resistance training (because if you do you'll burn through your carbs before you get to the resistance training) and don't exercise if you haven't eaten sometime during the 3-4 hours prior to your session.

If you really prefer to exercise in the morning on an empty stomach, you'll probably be okay assuming that you ate well the day before, but you have to realize that you're putting yourself at risk to burn muscle for fuel during exercise if you're working out at a moderate to high intensity level with no food in your system. If you choose to exercise on an empty stomach, be sure to have your bodyfat tested regularly to ensure that you're not losing muscle.

There are other reasons besides the risk of muscle loss that you don't want to do your resistance training immediately after cardio. If you start with cardio, you'll use the carbs available in your bloodstream for fuel rather than fat, since that's the easiest thing for your body to do. This means your weights workout will suffer since the carbs that are *required* for resistance training will already be burned through. Also, remember that bodyfat can't be broken down to be converted into glucose, so when you do cardio first followed by resistance training you'll never mobilize and burn off as much bodyfat as you would if you did the reverse. Even if you use all your available carbs during resistance training, it's perfectly fine (desirable, even) to go straight into cardio because your body will simply start burning bodyfat for fuel. On the contrary, if you do cardio first your body will have no choice but to burn muscle to provide the necessary glucose for your resistance training.

Even if you manage to not burn any muscle doing resistance training after cardio, your weights workout will definitely suffer when you've already burned through most of your carb stores. You won't be capable of lifting as hard or as heavy and therefore won't be stimulating your lean tissue to the same extent you could have if you had lifted first. That means you won't be burning as many calories with the resistance training, you won't be building as much muscle, you won't be raising your metabolism, and you'll also miss out on that post-calorie burn for which resistance training is king.

Another problem (we're almost done!) with doing cardio first is that you will tend to feel weaker and not perform as well by the time you get to the weight training, especially in the muscles that were involved during your cardio. For example, it's almost impossible to work as hard on your squats if you just finished running for 45 minutes. This is simply due to the fact that the muscles are fatigued, aside from the issue of whether there are enough carb stores left to fuel the activity.

However, if you do weights first followed by cardio, your cardio won't suffer much, if at all. This is because you can tap into the fat circulating in your bloodstream in addition to your bodyfat stores to get through the cardio, even if your glucose levels are low. Cardio also doesn't require much muscular strength, so it's not a big problem if your muscles are tired from lifting first. You'll still be able to perform your cardio with sufficient intensity after resistance training. To summarize, when you do cardio after weights (or at a completely different time) you get to experience the metabolism-boosting effects of both your resistance training and your cardio to the greatest extent.

If you go into almost any gym you will see some people doing exactly what I just said *not* to do – many people will do cardio first and then hit the weights. Why is that? It seems the main reason many people do cardio first is because they were told years ago that you don't want to lift weights when your muscles are cold because you can injure yourself. Therefore, it seemed to make sense to do cardio first. That advice was perpetuated before most people knew about the different fuel usage during cardio and resistance training.

The advice about not lifting with cold muscles *is* sound, but you can solve the cold-muscle problem simply by doing an easy cardio warm-up for 5-10 minutes before you hit the weights. Many people haven't caught up to speed with the new protocol because it's based on recent findings in exercise physiology. Some people actually *have* heard that it's better to do the weights first, but the people who hate doing cardio quite often can't resist doing it first simply to get it out of the way. That's a fine approach if you're willing to accept sub-optimal results with your bodyfat loss. But if you definitely want to lose as much fat as possible, you're going to *have* to do the weights first. And, if your primary goal is to gain muscle, you *absolutely* need to do the weights first. If your primary goal is muscle gain, consider doing cardio on an off day from the weights, if you do any at all.

On the other hand, if you're exercising because you know you should for health reasons or because you enjoy it and you don't care so much about the physique changes, do whatever you like – but keep in mind that you won't perform as well on the weights if you do cardio first. Although it might feel like cardio is harder to get through after the weights, your endurance shouldn't be affected very much when you do your cardio after your weight training.

Let me demonstrate with numbers how the comparison stacks up. Let's assume that you can perform at 100% with weights and 100% with cardio if you train them during separate workout sessions. If you do weights after cardio, your weights performance will be at about 60% (versus 100% if you weight-trained first or at a separate time). If you do cardio after weights, you'll probably perform at 90% (whereas if you did the cardio first or at a separate time you'd be at 100%). The saving grace for taking this 10% hit is that you'll burn more bodyfat when you do cardio after the weights.

As you can see, doing weights first or in a separate session is the way to go.

If you're an endurance athlete, your best bet is to do your resistance training at a separate time from your cardio if possible, since you may not be willing to accept even a 10% drop in performance during your cardio training (In case you're wondering, it is highly recommended that endurance athletes do a resistance-training routine at least twice per week to improve performance). If you have to do it all at once, I still recommend doing the weight-training first, because you'll be sacrificing too much if you choose the other option.

Racking up those miles assignment

1. If cardio isn't already part of your routine, consider scheduling a couple of sessions per week. If you've been doing cardio, look over your current regimen to see if it follows the recommendations you've read in this Strategy. Consider doing some additional reading or consult a trainer to find out which types of cardio are best for you. The sources listed in Reference E have sample cardio routines and some articles about cardio. Prescriptions for the optimal amount of cardio for each body type can be found in Reference D. Most trainers offer consultations for cardio training, which you can use to get personalized recommendations.

VI. Anti-Stagnant

Now that you've been successful in following an exercise routine, you need to start thinking about the future. Your exercise routine, like your body, is a work-in-progress. This section will teach you how to keep things interesting and how to stay healthy as an exerciser. You'll learn how to ensure that you continue to see results as you graduate to the status of an intermediate or advanced exerciser.

Strategy 25: Time to work out *again*?

Avoid getting bored with exercise

You need to change your workout routine periodically to keep from getting physically and mentally stale. For at least the first two months of your program, use a full-body resistance training routine plus cardio because that is what has been proven to yield the best results for beginners. Once you progress to the intermediate level, you'll need to decide whether you'd like to keep a full-body program or try a split routine. If fat loss is your primary goal, I recommend staying with a full-body workout, although split routines allow for more variety in training and can also work well. If you choose a split, realize that you still need to hit each body part at least twice per week for best results – for the natural lifter, volume of work for a particular body part can't make up for frequency. In other words, performing three sets for chest twice per week is better than performing six sets for chest during one workout but not hitting your chest again for a week.

One example of a split routine is to train chest, shoulders, and quads on day 1 and back, hamstrings and abs on day 2. That is an example of a 2-way split. A popular 3-way split is chest, shoulders and triceps on day 1, back and biceps on day 2, and legs and abs on day 3. There are countless variations that make physiological sense if you are familiar with exercise physiology and human anatomy and know how to design workout routines. A full-body routine is ideal for the natural lifter who wants to limit resistance training to three days per week. If you'd like to lift 4-6 days per week, a 2-way split will be your best bet, and if you're committed to six days of lifting a week you can choose a 3-way (Note: 5 or 6-way splits, common among bodybuilders, can be a good way to train if you're on steroids or andro. In those splits, you'd only target a bodypart once per week. For example, a 6-way split might have chest on Monday, back on Tuesday, quads and calfs on Wednesday, rest on Thursday, biceps and triceps on Friday, shoulders and hamstrings on Saturday, and abs on Sunday. For the natural lifter, this type of training is *not* the way to go. For the natural lifter, and some would argue for the steroid/andro user as well, it's ideal to hit each bodypart two or three times a week. Do three if you recover quickly and if you have the time – do two otherwise).

You don't necessarily have to change your entire program to incorporate variety into your workouts – there are ways to vary your training even if you keep the same exercises. Variables to manipulate include rep speed (both during the lifting and the lowering portion of an exercise), number of reps, and number of sets. You can add intensity sets like drop sets (doing a set with a challenging weight to near failure for 6-12 reps, then "dropping" or lowering the weight used but completing another 6-12 reps right away), supersets (two sets back-to-back that work opposing muscle groups), and compound sets (two sets back-to-back that work the same muscle group). Negatives and forced reps, described on page 212, are also types of intensity sets.

There are still other ways to incorporate variety into your training. You can try using dumbbells, barbells, cable machines, fitness balls, medicine balls, chin-up/dip bars, bodyweight exercises, cybex/nautilus machines, or hammer strength machines. Try some of your exercises one limb at a time (You'll be surprised by how hard this is! Use even less than half the weight you'd use for the "two-limbed" version the first time you try).

As you can see, there really is no excuse to get bored. And those examples I've given only cover resistance training. You can mix things up just as easily with cardio. Try outdoor activities such as cycling, walking, or running on different types of terrain. Try spending 5-10 minutes at a time on a cardio machine and switching machines 3-5 times during your workout. Challenge yourself to some of the programs on the cardio machines, or design your own workout using the manual program. Check out an aerobics class or two, or take your workout to the pool with swimming or water aerobics.

Circuit training is another good option if you get bored easily. You'll never have to do the same exercise two sets in a row, and you'll avoid monotony by throwing weights, cardio, and bodyweight exercises into the same exercise session. You'll have to stay on your toes to remember what comes next, and circuit training maximizes your time spent working out because it will improve your strength and your stamina during the same training session.

I have to work out *again*? assignment

1. Take the time to investigate new styles of training periodically, and experiment with new variations on basic exercises (consider a wide range of options such as Olympic-style lifting, kettlebells, bodyweight exercises, resistance bands, plyometrics, indoor cardio machines, stadium stairs, the outdoor track, a hiking trail, pool workouts, sports, martial arts, etc). The books, magazines, and websites listed in Resource E can give you even more ideas.

A trainer can help you design programs that include these variations. You should train for at least six weeks as a beginner with a basic program before you try anything fancy. In general, you'll see the fastest changes in body composition when you work out with weights and cardio rather than spend some of your workout time playing a sport or taking a group class where the activity is stop-and-start. However, if you find those options much more enjoyable than being in the gym, you'll be happier and more likely to stick with it, which means in the end you'll probably come out ahead. However, if you're the type that is motivated most by fast results that you can see in the mirror, you're better off staying in the gym and spending your time on the weights and cardio until you are close to where you want to be physically. Also, if your time is limited, you'll get the most bang for your buck time-wise when you stick with the weights and cardio. If you have plenty of time, are willing to be patient for results, and are looking to have fun while you train, consider sports, classes, and other more recreational types of exercise.

Although it's really only necessary to change your program every six weeks to continue enjoying steady progress, some people choose to perform a different workout every time they train. The main benefit to a strategy like this is that it staves off boredom by keeping workouts fun and interesting. It *is* a fact that people tend to work harder when something is new to them. When I work with a client multiple times per week, I usually incorporate lots of variety because it is more enjoyable for everyone and the client does generally see better results.

If you decide to keep the same routine for a full six weeks, your best bet will be to use a planned schedule of progressive resistance training. I use a version with my clients called "Progressive Resistance Cycle Training." This program consists of workout cycles during which you keep performing the same exercises, but never do the same workout two days in a row (instead, you vary the sets/reps/weight in a specific, incremental fashion). The progressive resistance program many of my clients have been using with great success is set up as 2-week blocks of six workouts each. Within these 2-week blocks, workout 1 is always the easiest and workout 6 is always the hardest.

In Progressive Resistance Cycle Training, the first 2-week block is followed by a second 2-week block during which you increase the weight a small amount for each of the six workouts. This means you both start and finish the second 2-week block using a heavier weight than you used in the first 2-week block. The same pattern is repeated for the third 2-week block. The three 2-week blocks are followed by one or two rest weeks during which you take time off from lifting. You can do cardio in conjunction with this resistance-training program if you like. After the first cycle (which takes 7 or 8 weeks to complete, including the rest period) you might continue with another 7 or 8-week cycle. By that time, however, you should be stronger and leaner than before.

Most people who try Progressive Resistance Cycle Training like it because they get to enjoy the "easy" workouts while at the same time get to anticipate the challenging ones coming up. Applying progressive resistance over time is scientifically proven to be the most effective way to increase muscle size and strength (12). As it turns out, the program is also great for maintaining lean body mass and metabolism while on a fat-loss diet. That's probably why "Progressive Resistance Cycle Training" has been one of my most popular programs to date. The great thing about Progressive Resistance Cycle Training is that, as long as you know the form for the handful of exercises you will use over the six-week period, your trainer can design your cycles and all you have to do is follow the workout cards that tell you how many sets and reps to do for each exercise on a given day. If you don't feel the need to use a trainer for motivation or additional form help, your trainer can even design the cycles over the phone or online. This will help to pare down training costs and means you won't have to worry about scheduling in-person workouts with a trainer, while still enjoying great results.

No matter which type of training you choose, be sure to investigate your options for varying your workouts. There is no reason to get bored with all the different training methods to try.

Strategy 26: Surprise, surprise!

Keep mixing things up

Every once in a while you should do something that's completely different from your usual routine. This will shock your body (in a good way) to rise to the new challenge and keep you from hitting a plateau. Perhaps most importantly, it will prevent you from getting bored with your workouts, which puts you at risk for losing interest in exercise.

Your body will adapt quickly to a specific movement. Once adaptation starts to occur, you become more efficient at performing the movement and don't "waste" (burn) as many calories exercising. Your muscles adapt rapidly at first, but then the adaptation starts to taper off. Instead of sticking to your usual routine as you slowly watch your progress grind to a halt, use your body's tendency toward rapid adaptation to your advantage by introducing new movements on a regular basis.

Really get creative – don't limit yourself to switching between a barbell chest press and a dumbbell chest press and try to call that "variety!" Experiment with many different things. For example, the two basic variations for working chest are the flat bench barbell chest press and the flat bench dumbbell chest press. Try doing those presses on an incline and decline bench as well. Also try flat, incline, and decline dumbbell flys. Experiment with different types of push-ups, a machine chest press, a medicine ball chest toss, the high-pulley cable fly, the low-pulley cable fly, dips, and the pec dec.

In the cardio department, bring your treadmill jog outdoors once in a while, and consider working your way up to sprints or trail running. Give the stairmaster a break and run the bleachers at your high school stadium. Take a bike ride. Try a new aerobics class, even if you're afraid of looking silly because you don't know the steps. Just go to the back of the room and have fun learning. You'll be surprised how fast the time passes when you try something new, and many times you'll end up working out longer than you had planned without meaning to. You'll know that you've had a great workout both physically and mentally because all of a sudden you'll realize that you feel pretty wiped out, in a good way.

Do you remember that rush of adrenaline you felt as a kid when you tried something new? You can have that feeling again. It will make your workouts so much more productive and exciting. Consider joining a sports team or a martial arts class. By expanding your horizons, at the very least you'll get another workout in, and at best you'll find a new activity that you absolutely love!

Surprise, surprise! assignment

1.   After you've familiarized yourself with some of your options for working out, schedule some different workouts into your day planner, preferably involving at least one new activity or one new workout venue a month. You might vary the actual exercises or just the order in which you do them. You might try working out at home rather than at the gym, or try working out with an exercise buddy (have a "routine swap" day with someone who works out at your gym – you each do the other's usual workout for the day). Buy a day pass to a gym in the next town and sample the different machines.

   If you don't plan for these variations, you might end up following your typical routine for months on end. Of course, the most important thing is to simply keep exercising in some form or another, but you will get better results and enjoy your time much more when you take the initiative to switch up your routine. And, anything that's worth doing is worth planning for to be *sure* it gets done. Take control of how you live your life and how you work out!

Strategy 27: Strain to Gain

How to push through your exercise comfort zone

Your effort level is ultimately what will dictate your results. Your workouts provide the stimulus that leads your body to change. If they aren't challenging enough, your body won't have a need to adapt. Your body will adapt for the better as long as your intensity level in the gym is sufficient, provided of course that you train smart. Training smart means taking rest days and easy days in addition to having days when you push yourself more. If you exercise your body using focus and discipline, it will take on a lean and toned look. On the other hand, if you're lazy with your workouts, your body will show the world.

Certain mental techniques can be helpful for improving performance during your workouts. I'll explain a few of them now.

1. The "mini-set" trick. On days when you are working on the brink of your pain threshold, 8 or 12 reps can seem like a long way away. It is easier psychologically to count in smaller groups – say, three groups of 4. So, in this case instead of counting to 12 you'd count to 4 three times. It might sound hokey, but mind games like this can help you achieve at a higher level. Your mind will sometimes fight with you when you go beyond your usual number of reps with a given weight. Once your brain starts protesting, your perception of physical discomfort increases because your mind tells your muscles that they should expect to be tired and hurting. The "mini-set" trick helps you fight against that perception. Another related technique is to count *down from* 12, rather than *up to* 12. It really does make the set seem more manageable, especially toward the end.

2. The "rest on the horizon" trick. Another tip is to use rest days coming up in your schedule as incentive to push yourself harder while you're "under the bar." It's easier to work hard if you know you'll get to enjoy a break soon. Plus, you'll feel better on your rest days if you know that you pushed yourself during your workouts. You can force yourself to "earn" your rest days or easy days by working at a high intensity level on the tougher days. After all, you want to have something to rest *from* so that your time off won't be for nothing.

3. The "last set" trick. If it's your last set for the day, or even your last set for a muscle group, challenge yourself to continue until you hit absolute muscular failure. You'll find it easier to train to complete exhaustion of the muscle if you know you won't have to do another set for that muscle. The pain will be easier to deal with because you'll know "it won't get any worse than this" and soon you'll get to relax.

4. The "one more" trick. Once you hit your target number of reps, challenge yourself to push out "one more." See how many "one mores" you can squeak out.

5. The "social pressure" trick. Most people find that they push themselves harder when they're being watched. Whether you're being watched by a training partner, a personal trainer, or even just the group of people around you lifting at the gym, you'll find that you're more likely to push yourself when there are other people around, especially on days when you don't have a ton of energy. Everyone tends to want to put his best foot forward in front of others – this is a basic pattern of social behavior. You'll also get to enjoy the positive feedback from others when you do well, which most people find motivating. On the other hand, if you tend to be more internally than externally motivated, you might find that keeping a detailed training log helps you push yourself more than anything else because you will get a rush out of seeing a new personal best marked down in your log.

Keep in mind that high-intensity workouts should be limited to, at most, one or two sessions per week. Many injuries and cases of overtraining occur when people spend too many workouts pushing themselves beyond their recovery capabilities. Make sure that you train at varying intensity levels, whether you schedule them ahead of time or just decide from workout to workout. Some people like to plan each day's workout ahead of time, while others prefer to decide what to do based on how they feel day-to-day.

If you are highly sensitive to changes in mood and energy level, basing your workout on how you feel may be your best bet. The day-to-day, "wing it" technique also allows you to take advantage of high-energy days by working harder, while allowing you to take it easier on low-energy days. Just be careful that you don't justify avoiding the harder workouts all the time because you don't "feel" like it. If you *always* seem to have low-energy days, you might have to push yourself to work hard anyway to get the results you want. Most of the time, working out harder actually improves your energy levels overall, so hopefully low energy won't be a problem for long!

Some people prefer to vary their intensity *within* each workout rather than *between* workouts. In this case, you'd work some of the muscles you hit in a given workout harder and some easier. The next time you hit those muscle groups, you'd switch it up and do the reverse.

If you're willing to commit to six weeks of workouts with a 3-day per week schedule, you can use progressive resistance techniques such as Progressive Resistance Cycle Training as explained in Strategy 25 and Reference C. If you follow a plan like this, you'll know that your overall intensity is at the right level to optimize progress.

As I have already noted in previous Strategies, at the intermediate and advanced fitness level almost everyone's body resists building muscle and shedding fat at the same time. Exercisers at this level progress the fastest when they dedicate months at a time to a particular goal, such as building muscle or losing fat. These are sometimes called "bulking" and "cutting" cycles and the main difference between the two plans is calorie intake and amount of cardio in the training schedule.

Bulking cycles are characterized by resistance training in the low, medium, and high-rep ranges (anything from 3-15 reps per set), little or no cardio, and eating above-maintenance calories (being in a calorie surplus). The goal for a bulking cycle is to gain weight, and preferably more muscle than fat.

Cutting cycles are characterized by resistance training in the medium and high-rep ranges (8-15 reps), more cardio, and eating below-maintenance calories (running a calorie deficit). A common misconception is that you can "bulk up" just from lifting heavy weights. The reality is that you also need to be eating above-maintenance calories to put on size. The reason dieters should shy away from low-rep training in the 3-8-rep range is because dieters are more susceptible to injuries. While heavy weights shouldn't cause problems if you're maintaining your weight or gaining weight, dieters tend to get injured much more easily. This is due to the fact that those eating fewer calories have less fluid in their bodies to lubricate joints and support muscles, a reduced ability to recover due to a shortage of nutrients, and lower energy levels due to a reduced calorie intake. Even when a dieter stays in the optimal calorie deficit (which is approximately 500 calories per day) these "problems" still exist. These "problems" are a result of running an energy deficit, and, if you're dieting successfully, *by definition* you're running an energy deficit. If you diet smart by keeping the optimal energy deficit and dieting in blocks of 6-8 weeks before taking at least two weeks off to eat at or above maintenance calories, you will minimize the problems inherent to dieting, but you can never eliminate them completely.

The body responds best when your diet and workouts are both dialed in to achieve a single goal. As you work toward that goal, your workout intensity should be varied in a systematic fashion for best results. Progressive resistance on the body systems over time is what will get you the results you're after, not only with resistance training but also with the volume and intensity of cardio and with your diet.

For example, let's assume that your first month of a cardio routine involves three 20-minute sessions per week of steady-pace jogging. To use the progressive resistance principle, the next month you'd want to "up the ante." This might mean moving to three 30-minute sessions per week. Then you'd "up" it again to three 40-minute sessions per week the following month. This increase over time, provided that your calorie intake stays consistent, will encourage your body to shed fat. This type of systematic increase has a more powerful effect on your body than if you were to do three 30-minute sessions per week during the entire three-month period, even though the average amount of time spent on exercise is the same in both instances. In this example, after the three months of progressive increase with cardio you might switch your cardio activity and use the same progressive buildup with the new activity.

This "up-the-ante" technique is effective with diet as well. Start a diet by cutting back some on calories and junk food here and there, and progressively get stricter as your weight loss cycle continues. (Note: This is the opposite approach to going on a "crash" diet!) Then you can take a break and go back for another cycle if needed.

Systematic changes in diet and training make the whole process of getting into shape much faster and much easier. What's nice about using systematic changes is that on any given day you'll only be doing a little more than you're used to. You never have to face a huge change, yet you still get great results – and in many cases, better results than if you try to work at your limit every day. You're also less likely to get bored because you'll always be changing something about your routine depending on where you are in your "cycle." You'll be less likely to get injured or overtrained too, because you will have plenty of "easy" days and rest time thrown into the mix.

The major downside to using progressive resistance with diet and training is that it works best when you stick to a regimented plan, which doesn't leave many allowances for times when life gets in the way of the gym (including illness and injury). If you break the pattern of the progressive increase, your results won't be quite as good. Still, even if your cycles aren't completed in perfect progressive form, you still should see acceptable results if you do the best you can under the circumstances. Another potential downside to using strict progressive resistance is that your energy level and motivation might be out-of-sync with your training program at times. In other words, you might feel strong and energetic on an "easy" day and have to hold back, but when you get to the "hard" day you might not have it in you to push yourself.

To sum up this discussion, you have two options for training most effectively: One is to use cycles of training with progressive resistance, and the other is to have easy, medium, and hard days that are placed randomly in your schedule. You'll need to weigh the pros and cons to decide what seems best for you at this point. Keep in mind that your intensity can still be varied systematically even if you use a random schedule – everything across the board should be at a higher level as you become more conditioned and as you move through your 8 weeks of training following your rest week. For instance, when you're starting out an easy day might be walking at 3.0 m.p.h. on flat ground and a hard day might be walking at 3.5 m.p.h. with a 5% incline. Six months later, the incline walk might be an easy day for you, and your hard day might involve jogging at 5.5 m.p.h. with a 3% incline. On the resistance-training end, after a rest week you might try lifting just 75% of the amount of weight you'd normally use. By the eighth week of training, try to hit personal bests in most of your lifts. If you're not sure you want or need to take a rest week, you'll probably change your mind once you read Strategy 29.

Strain to Gain assignment

1. You'll probably need to do some research or consult a trainer who is well-versed in progressive resistance techniques if you're interested in setting up cycles of diet and training. Only consider using strict cycles for your training if you're willing to follow specific instructions and won't mind the regimentation and lack of spontaneity. Cycle training will be a good choice if you're determined to achieve quicker results than you would generally have by simply working out and eating well. Hiring a trainer to work with you on a regular basis is another great way to ensure that you push through your exercise comfort zone at times.

2. Try some of the intensity tricks from this Strategy, but keep in mind that you shouldn't work out with maximum intensity every time you train. This will do more harm than good. You should, however, vary your intensity so that 1-2 workouts a week (one resistance training workout and/or one cardio workout) are performed at or near your maximum level. This is the frequency that will allow you to maximize the benefits of high-intensity training without draining your energy and harming your health in the process. At this frequency of high-intensity work you should find yourself looking forward to the challenge without feeling like you're dreading yet another brutal training session. You should be able to stay physically and psychologically fresh and remain happy and healthy and while enjoying steady progress.

Strategy 28: Handle with care

How to treat your body right

Stretching and taking care of injuries are very important for your physical well-being. The stress of exercise makes it even more critical that you take care of your body and muscles. A good flexibility program hits all the muscles of the body, with extra focus on areas where your muscles are tighter. Generally, there is no need to stretch immediately before your workout. The only time it is preferable to stretch before exercise is when you are about to participate in a flexibility-intensive activity such as gymnastics, martial arts or dance, or if a physical therapist has prescribed stretching prior to an activity due to an injury you've sustained.

You will, however, perform best during your workout and minimize your risk for injury when you do some gentle cardio as a warm-up. This prepares your muscles and joints for the workout to come. The warm-up should consist of 5-10 minutes of easy cardio such as walking, marching in place, or slow stair-stepping. The purpose of the warm-up is to elevate your heart rate, raise your body temperature, bring blood to your muscles, and lubricate your joints.

Some people like to stretch their muscles while they're resting in between sets. This is okay to do – but avoid stretching the muscles that you are about to work. Stretching weakens a muscle for a couple of minutes afterward, which means it can interfere with your lifting strength. However, it's perfectly fine to stretch a muscle that you won't be using for the next few minutes. This won't interfere with your workout at all.

The best time for a complete stretching program is immediately following any type of workout. After a workout your muscles will be warm and there will be plenty of blood flowing through them, which makes it easier to stretch and reduces the likelihood that you'll pull a muscle or tendon. Move slowly into each stretch and hold it at the point where you feel a strong tug. You *don't* want to push so far that you feel a sharp twinge or pain. If this happens, you'll know you have gone too far and should take the cue to back off. Your muscles won't relax and limber up if you stretch them too aggressively – muscles clamp up as a protective mechanism when they are overstretched, which works against your purpose for stretching in the first place.

If you aren't motivated to stretch for the sake of injury prevention or simply because it feels good, you might be motivated to do it knowing that it will make you stronger. It's a fact that exercisers who perform a stretching routine along with a resistance-training regimen get stronger faster than those who skip the stretching.

You should hold each stretch for 20-30 seconds. For supertight areas, repeat the stretch for a total of two or three rounds. There are many books, magazines, and websites that you can refer to if you don't know how to stretch all the muscles in your body. Personal trainers and physical therapists can show you how to stretch most effectively, and some will stretch your muscles for you while you relax. When someone stretches you it is generally more effective, but you can still do a great job on your own if you know how to stretch the right way. There are also some neat techniques for stretching that can help with chronic tightness and injuries and allow you to attain a higher degree of flexibility than you could with just a basic stretching program. The most important thing, however, is to get into a regular stretching routine, even if you reserve just five minutes for stretching twice a week after workouts.

Injury prevention and rehabilitation will become an issue for almost every exerciser at some point. The best tip for injury prevention is to listen to your body. Exercise should result in a somewhat uncomfortable tension in the muscles, but never a sharp pain. A sharp pain or twinge while working out, especially in the joints, is not a good sign. If this occurs, try using less weight, or stop the exercise altogether. You may or may not be able to find a substitute exercise that works the same area without causing the injury to flare up. If your injury was minor, after a week pain-free you can try again to see if you can lift without pain. There is a lot of trial and error involved in resistance training and with exercising in general.

A physical therapist will need to step in if your injuries persist. Also, keep in mind that it is always preferable to exercise without pain, especially since there is usually some substitute exercise or activity that won't bother the area. For those reasons, I'm not going to discuss injury treatment in detail. I'll just give you a quick overview on the treatment of minor injuries.

If you experience pain while working out, you need to rest the injured area until the pain subsides. Anti-inflammatories are helpful to reduce swelling. However, don't try to exercise the injured area while taking anti-inflammatories or other pain-relievers, because you might do further damage and not know it until later on.

Ice packs and heat pads are the most common treatments for injuries related to physical activity. It's important that you know which treatment to use and how to use it for effective self-treatment of minor injuries (13).

Ice is the most common treatment for acute injuries. If you have a recent injury (sustained within the last 48 hours) accompanied by swelling, you should use ice treatment. Ice packs can help minimize swelling associated with an injury.

Ice packs are typically used after injuries such as an ankle sprain. Applying an ice pack early and often for the first 48 hours will help minimize swelling. Decreasing the swelling around an injury will help control the pain. Apply ice treatments for no longer than 20 minutes at a time. Too much ice can do harm and can even cause frostbite.

Ice treatments may also be used for chronic conditions such as overuse injuries. For chronic injuries, you'll want to ice the injured area *after* activity. This will help control the inflammatory response. Never ice a chronic injury before activity.

Heat treatments should be used for chronic conditions before activity to help relax and loosen tissues and to stimulate blood flow to the area, which aids in healing. Only use heat treatments on chronic conditions, such as overuse injuries, *before* participating in the bothersome activity. Do not use heat on an acute injury.

A heating pad or a hot, wet towel can be used for heat treatments. When using heat treatments, be careful to use just moderate heat for a limited period of time (in order to avoid burns). Never leave heating pads turned on for long periods of time, and never leave a heating pad unattended if it's plugged in, even if it's not turned on.

If the pain persists in spite of rest and treatment, try a substitute exercise or activity. If the area continues to hurt no matter which exercise you use, you'll need to see a physical therapist or an orthopedic for specific advice and treatment. Don't allow a personal trainer to give anything beyond general advice on injury treatment unless he has a certification, license, or degree in sports medicine, injury rehabilitation, or physical therapy.

Handle with care assignment

1. Learn how to stretch all the major muscle groups in the body. You might look to books and websites on stretching for guidance. Most trainers and physical therapists will design personalized stretching regimens.

2. Decide how you'd like to work on your flexibility. Some people practice gymnastics, dance, martial arts, or yoga to learn stretches and improve their flexibility. The quickest route to gaining flexibility is to dedicate 10-15 minutes to stretching after your workout three days per week. Simply hold the basic stretches for 20-30 seconds each, making sure to target all parts of the body. If you aren't willing to commit that amount of time to stretching, set aside just five minutes twice per week. You'll probably notice that you feel much better and start getting stronger (since a more flexible muscle is a stronger muscle), and at that point you may be motivated to devote more time to stretching. If not, you'll still enjoy the benefits of stretching when you spend just ten minutes per week on flexibility. Plan your stretching time into your total workout time so that you don't find excuses to put it off.

Strategy 29: Sit down al ready!

Why rest is crucial to achieving the body you want

Rest and recovery deserve just as much consideration as your workouts if you're serious about getting in shape, particularly when your program includes resistance training. To understand why, a simplified physiology lesson is in order.

Your muscles must contract in order to lift a weight or even just to move a part of your body. When a muscle contracts, it becomes shorter and firmer to the touch as the microscopic muscle fibers slide over one another. With a sufficient stimulus, such as that which occurs when lifting a heavy weight, these muscle fibers actually pull apart, causing trauma at the micro-level. Your body responds to this stress by rebuilding the bridges between the muscle fibers to return things to normal. The reason weight-training makes you stronger is because after the initial disruption your body repairs itself to be slightly stronger than it was before so that next time it will be able to manage the stimulus more effectively. What you need to remember is that the building-up part happens *between*, not *during*, workouts.

In other words, what you do *outside* the gym is just as important as what you do *in* the gym. Another thing you need to realize is that your body operates as a system, not as a collection of unrelated parts. If you apply stress to just one group of muscles, your entire system still takes an impact. This alludes to the discussion about generalized stress on the central nervous system in previous Strategies. Even if you provide enough rest for each individual muscle, if you do too much work overall your central nervous system will become overloaded. And if you don't allow your body sufficient time for repair and rebuilding, you will fail to recover and become stronger. You will also place yourself at high risk for developing chronic injuries, chronic fatigue, and eventually, overtraining syndrome.

Overtraining syndrome occurs when you've been training too much or too hard for too long. This can be the result of too much working out, not enough recovery, or a combination of the two. For example, a person who works out ten hours a week will generally be at a higher risk for overtraining than someone who works out five hours a week. Also, someone who works part-time and sleeps eight hours a night can generally handle a greater workout volume and intensity than someone who works full-time and only gets five hours of sleep a night. However, there are also individual differences in how quickly someone reaches the state of overtraining, regardless of lifestyle. You simply might need more or less recovery than the average person. There's really no way to know which category you fall into until you start an exercise routine and keep your eye out for symptoms, which I will describe shortly.

"Overtraining" in the short-term is known as overreaching. Overreaching may be the result of something as simple as pushing yourself just a little too hard during a workout, or it may be a case of not getting enough rest across a week of training. Overreaching is a precursor to full-blown overtraining syndrome.

The true state of overtraining takes time to occur, but unfortunately by the time it gets serious it will require some bigtime recovery. The damage won't be easily undone at that point. To prevent overtraining, be sure to work within your limits. Besides following the training guidelines as detailed throughout this book, it's important that you listen to your body. If you begin to feel lethargic, unmotivated, experience an appetite increase or decrease, feel depressed, have sleeping difficulties, or stop making progress in the gym, you may be overreaching, and therefore are a prime candidate for overtraining.

Other symptoms of doing too much include headaches, lowered resistance to common illness, slowed healing, pain in the muscles and joints, and an increase in anxiety level. If you begin experiencing these symptoms, "quit" while you're ahead. Take some time to rest, and then ease back into a reasonable workout schedule. You'll feel rejuvenated and hopefully will be able to avoid illness, injury, and burnout.

Everyone varies in the amount of rest they need. You'll discover the amount that's best for you by trial and error, always keeping the general recommendations in mind. The amount of rest you require will depend partly on how much you have going on in your life at the time. Be aware that a beginner will not be able to handle the same workload as an experienced exerciser.

However, the fact is that beginners don't even *need* the same workload to make substantial progress. A beginner can make progress training as infrequently as twice per week, performing one set per exercise for all the major muscle groups. This type of routine might consist of 6-12 exercises, or 12-24 sets per week. At the opposite extreme, many elite athletes train nearly every day, and sometimes multiple times per day (using split workouts for the most part). The average person who has been working out regularly will fall somewhere in between, opting to train weights and cardio 2-4 times a week for about 30 minutes each.

A good rule of thumb is that, as frequency of workouts goes up, volume of each workout should go down. For example, if you train twice per week, it makes sense to use a full body routine with about 20 sets in total at a high average intensity. If you train 5-6 times per week, you'll need to use a shorter workout and target different muscles on different days. For best results, hit each major muscle group 2-3 times per week. This is the most effective way to train as a natural lifter (the rules are different for people using andro or steroids). That means, if you lift four days per week, you'll want to hit half of your body on day 1 and the other half on day 2, and then repeat day 1 and day 2 during your workout week for a total of four training sessions per week.

When you follow the recommendation to hit the same muscle multiple times per week, it's important that you vary the intensity of your workouts. For instance, if you're squatting three days per week, train with heavy weight and low reps one day, use medium weight and medium reps another day, and go light with higher reps on the third day. In addition to varying the intensity, it helps with recovery and promotes complete muscle development to use different exercises and hit the muscle from different angles within your workout week. For instance, if you're hitting chest twice per week, it makes sense to do the flat bench press and the incline dumbbell press one day and push-ups and the high-pulley cable chest fly another day.

Now that I've covered rest/recovery within your workout schedule, you might be wondering if time off from exercise is necessary. The answer is yes! You should take at least 7-10 days off from lifting every 8-12 weeks. If you are an experienced lifter and work out with heavy weights, your best bet is to take 10-14 days off every eight weeks.

It actually takes about 4 weeks away from the gym to lose a significant amount of muscle tissue, so these 1 to 2-week rests won't cause you to lose muscle or gain any appreciable amount of fat. On the contrary, by allowing for full system recovery you will actually set yourself up to make faster progress than you would if you trained straight through. Besides, there is a psychological benefit to taking time off. When it's time to get back into your workout routine, you will enjoy newfound vigor for what seemed monotonous before. If you'd like, you may continue some easy or moderate-pace cardio during your "off" weeks, although you should refrain from sprints, hills or other high-intensity cardio sessions.

Sleep is also fundamental to fitness success. Expect your performance in the gym to be impaired after a few nights of poor sleep. In addition to reduced performance, your body's hormonal makeup shifts when you haven't had enough rest. This means the work you *do* get done in the gym won't be as effective. The stress hormones your body releases when you're sleep-deprived leads to a loss of lean tissue, a gain in fat mass, a sluggish metabolism, and slow recovery. Also, your immune system is compromised when you don't sleep enough, meaning that whatever viruses are lurking in your environment will be accepted more easily by your body.

The critical importance of sleep to your progress is another reason why it might not be in your best interest to use any type of stimulant, including those found in most diet pills. Watch the medications you're taking too, because many over-the-counter and prescription drugs list insomnia as a side effect. Not taking any pills? The root of insomnia quite often lies in poor sleep habits. Here are "Ten Tips for Better Sleep" from the Better Sleep Council (14):

1. Give yourself "permission" to go to bed when it's getting late.
2. Unwind early in the evening.
3. Develop a sleep ritual.
4. Keep regular sleeping hours.
5. Create a restful place to sleep.
6. Sleep on a comfortable, supportive mattress and foundation.
7. Exercise regularly.
8. Cut down on stimulants.
9. Don't smoke.
10. Reduce alcohol intake.

For more advice, go to www.bettersleep.org where you can download a free copy of the Better Sleep Guide, or request a free copy from the Better Sleep Council, P.O. Box 19534, Alexandria, VA 22320.

Sit down already! assignment

1. Check your program to make sure that it has the appropriate amount of rest built in. Make sure to include rest days and easy days within each workout week, as well as full weeks with no workouts at all.

2. If you don't get enough sleep or don't sleep well, start searching for causes and potential solutions.

3. If you've covered all of the above and still want to improve your recovery from workouts, consider these "active recovery" or "restoration" tools. They include:

- Massage
- Easy to moderate cardio after resistance training or on alternate days
- Warm/hot baths, or periods of warm/hot immersion alternated with cool/cold immersion, such as going from a hot tub to a pool
- Various types of stretching, including active mobility such as tai chi and yoga
- Good nutrition with sufficient calorie intake
- Supplementation geared toward improving recovery and maintaining good health, such as a basic multivitamin/mineral, EFA supplementation, extra antioxidants, extra zinc/magnesium/calcium, glucosamine chondroitin, green tea extract, and ginsing
- Attention to psychological needs in training, such as variety, fun, and setting realistic goals

Strategy 30: Congratulate yourself!

How to completely enjoy and appreciate all that you've accomplished

If you aren't able to step back from all this work to congratulate yourself and feel proud of your accomplishments, what's the point? There will always be someone stronger, leaner, smarter, richer, or prettier than you, but you are doing yourself a disservice by comparing yourself to a theoretical ideal.

Strive to be your best, but don't berate yourself if you fall short. If you find yourself doing so, you might want to reevaluate your goals and decide what is really important to you. If you decide you're happy to be working out three days a week and want to forget about six, that's fine. On the other hand, if you decide that getting in peak shape is very important to you, you'll need to recommit yourself to going for it all. Either way, hopefully you can learn to enjoy the process rather than just be concerned with the end result. That way, you will never lose and you will never have a truly bad day.

This book is about success – and that means achieving what *you* want for your life. There is no reason to define fitness success as 10% body fat with ripped abs. If you'd like to try to achieve that, chances are you can – although it will almost always require a lot of hard work and a good amount of sacrifice in other areas of your life. Personally, I admire someone who is reasonably fit and healthy and has a full life more than I do someone who works out obsessively but doesn't leave time for anything else.

If your goal is to be the proud owner of a healthy, fit body, and you achieve that goal, even sans ripped abs – well, as far as I'm concerned you have achieved success, and I will be ecstatic for you!

Congratulate yourself! assignment

1. Enjoy.

VII. Reference

Reference A.
"The 10 Tricks You Need to Know to Eat Right, one person at a time"

Let's face it – eating right can be a pain, especially if you don't have anyone to cook for, or if you need to prepare some extra meals just for yourself. Whether you live alone or cook for a family, there will be times when you're watching what you eat that you'll need to cook a healthy meal just for you. Not to worry, though – once you learn the tricks of the trade, you will be shocked by how easy it is. Here are my ten best tips:

1. Buy food in bulk. Most people aren't too fond of going grocery shopping. If this is the case for you, buy enough food for at least a week to make each trip worth your while. Stock up if you find sales on frozen, packaged, or canned goods. You'll increase your chances of staying with your diet if you make sure to never run out of healthy, nutritious foods. If you're running low on supplies, you're much more likely to eat poorly, skip meals, or go out to eat, so be sure to keep the good stuff around all the time. Buying in bulk will usually help you save money too, although you need to be careful – sometimes bulk sizes are actually more expensive because the store figures that you won't notice (they know *that customers know* it's usually cheaper to buy in bulk). Check unit prices for an accurate cost comparison. Also, be sure that you have adequate storage space before you buy (or enough hungry people to feed), because no matter how inexpensive the food is, you're not saving anything if it spoils!

2. Prepare food in bulk. You'll find that preparing food in bulk saves a lot of time. For instance, you can boil a box of pasta or rice and keep it in the refrigerator, adding it to meals and dishes as needed. The fastest way to prepare chicken healthfully (a diet staple if there ever was one) is to buy a package of frozen boneless chicken breasts and boil them in a big pot. If you prefer, you can grill them for a short time afterward, or chop them up for stir-fry. Once the chicken is cooked, decide whether you have more than you will eat in the next four days. You can store any extra in the freezer. You might prefer to separate the meat before you freeze it so you can just cook enough for four days and won't have to re-freeze cooked meat. Leave the chicken in the refrigerator so you'll have a protein source that's ready to be added to various dishes. You can also add sauces and seasonings as you prepare your meals. All you'll have to do is grab those ingredients and a chicken breast, mix it together and throw it in the microwave. You can hard-boil eggs and grill or broil steak or fish ahead of time in the same manner. Also, any time you make a casserole, stir-fry, or soup, prepare extra and refrigerate or freeze it so you'll have a quick, easy meal option on hand.

3.   Frozen vegetables. These can be a godsend when you're crunched for time. In general, they are just as nutritious as fresh veggies. In some cases, canned and frozen vegetables are actually *more* nutritious because they are usually packaged at the peak of freshness, whereas there's no guarantee how long the "fresh" veggies have been lying around. Buy a few of your favorites each time you shop. Frozen veggies can be quickly prepared a serving at a time, which is about 1/3 bag for one person (this actually "counts" as 2 servings of veggies according to nutritionists). Cook an entire bag if you're feeding two or three people. Steam them in the microwave (just put them in a dish as is – you don't need to cover the dish, add water, or use plastic wrap) and they come out great. Usually 5-10 minutes will do the trick. Then you can add any oil or seasonings you want as well as some protein such as cut-up chicken and you'll have a low-calorie but tasty and nutritious meal.

4.   Pre-bagged salad and canned or packaged soups. These are a couple of wonderful modern conveniences. Salads are great to bring to work or on the road. Again, always add protein to your veggies, and some healthy fats from olive oil or nuts is a good addition too. It's true that pre-bagged salads cost more per pound, but they are super-convenient and will reduce the amount of food you lose to spoilage if you are the only one eating it. Instead of pre-bagged salad, you might opt for the grocery store's salad bar so that you can pick and choose the ingredients. The salad bar also makes for a quick, healthy lunch on the road. What's great about the salad bar is that there are usually a couple of choices for lean protein in addition to all the veggies. If you're considering canned or packaged soups, look for the "healthy" versions that are reduced-sodium and relatively low-fat and also contain some protein. Fruit is another nutritious option that is easy to store and transport.

5.   Rice, noodles, and cereal. Rice and noodles can be cooked ahead and left in the refrigerator for easy meal-making. Oatmeal makes a great "meal" when you want something quick and hot. Use "old fashioned" or whole oats, which aren't as processed as the "quick" oats and still cook within minutes in the microwave. Add water or skim milk and cook your oats in the microwave for 2-4 minutes. You might want to add fruit and cinnamon, peanut butter and a sweetener, or other things to liven up the taste of your oatmeal. Whole-grain, higher-protein and high-fiber cereals such as Kashi are also a good source of nutritious complex carbs. Just be sure to check the sugar and fat content, because some of the "healthy" cereals sneak in these extras, which will bump up the calorie content.

6. **Oils and seasonings.** I've already explained what you are to do with these guys. Always have the healthier ones on hand. Olive oil and most other oils will keep just fine if you store them in a cool, dark place. You can stock up on most of these staples on sale, although be careful with flax oil, which is becoming quite popular among those interested in health food. Flaxseed and flax oil are extremely nutritious and are two of the best sources of essential fatty acids, but those EFAs can be destroyed when heated to a high temperature or exposed to light. Therefore, flaxseed and flax oil should be stored in dark packaging in the refrigerator.

7. **Microwave.** I've already explained many of the uses for the microwave when eating healthy for one. You can re-heat your pre-made meals quickly one serving at a time in the microwave (unless you like cold food, in which case you get to save a step). I love the fact that I can throw something in the microwave and go check my email or do a few chores and find that my meal is ready for me within a few minutes. You can even cook some foods from scratch in the microwave. Want a potato? Just wash it in the sink, pierce it a few times with a fork, and put it in the microwave for about ten minutes. You can also cook chicken tenders in the microwave for a quick source of lean protein. Take a few raw strips of chicken, add ¼ cup of water, cover the dish, and "fire up" the microwave. You'll need to cook the tenders about 8 minutes for ¼ pound, 12 minutes for ½ pound, and 20 minutes for one pound. Make sure the poultry turns completely white, and once it does, let the meat cook for a few more minutes just to make sure it's done. Check labels for cooking instructions on your favorite food products, as some might have a microwave-cooking method you can try.

8. **Storage.** Hopefully you realize the importance of this concept by now! The two issues at hand are cupboard/pantry storage and

refrigerator/freezer storage. Invest in a good set of plastic containers in a variety of sizes. Cereal and other dry foods stay much better in plastic containers (no, folding the plastic bag inside the box isn't doing much), especially if you don't expect to finish it within a week. The containers will also come in handy for storing meals that you've prepared ahead. You will save money and reduce waste by using washable containers to store cooked food rather than wrapping it in plastic or foil.

9.   Meal replacement bars and drinks. These should not be used to the exclusion of "real" food, but 1-2 servings a day can go a long way toward helping round out your diet. One reason they can be a good choice is that you can select the bar or shake that matches the macronutrient profile you're looking for. You can find anything from high-protein, low-carb bars and shakes to high-carb "energy" products, or even "balanced" products that contain a moderate amount of carbs, protein, and fat. There are snack-sized choices and meal sized choices, as well as products that are formulated specifically for post-workout nutrition. Since post-workout is the most critical time of day for getting the proper nutrition, consider using one of the post-workout nutrition products.

It's critical that you get sufficient carbs and protein into your body for optimal recovery after resistance training, and the faster those nutrients hit your bloodstream the better. Don't worry about any specific nutrition regimen after cardio if your primary goal is fat loss – just eat your regular meal or snack whenever it's time. However, if you're training for an endurance competition and you want to maximize performance for your next training session, you should have some carbs along with a little bit of protein immediately after training. This will ensure that you have muscle glycogen available for your next training session.

After your resistance training, you need at least 1/3 gram of carbs per pound of bodyweight, and half as many grams of protein. For example, a 150-pound person would need at least 50 grams of carbs and 25 grams of protein. Both carbs and protein contain 4 calories per gram, so this is equivalent to 200 calories of carbs (50 grams x 4 calories per gram) and 100 calories of protein (25 grams x 4 calories per gram). Try to keep your post-workout meal or snack low in fat because fat will delay gastric emptying, and immediately following your workout you want those nutrients to hit your bloodstream as soon as possible.

A 150-pound person might fulfill these post-workout nutrition requirements by consuming a post-workout nutrition product containing 50 grams of carbs, 25 grams of protein, and 4 grams of fat. MET-Rx makes a great post-workout bar called "Big 100." If you want to use a bar, that's the brand I recommend both for taste and nutrition. Shakes usually contain higher-quality protein and carbs and therefore are preferable to bars if you have an option. Another reason you might want to opt for a shake is that protein powder is less expensive than bars, although the pre-mixed shakes you can buy a single-serving at a time are just as expensive as bars.

The most economical way to get your post-workout nutrition is to have a drink mixed with 100% whey protein powder plus almost any high-carb food as a snack after your workout. Optimum Nutrition's 100% Whey protein powder stirred into a cup of milk will do the trick, and be sure to add a high-carb food such as a small bagel to bump up the carb-count in your post-workout snack. Most of the sports nutrition brands carry a post-workout shake that includes the carbs you need along with the protein, which is more convenient than having to add your own carbs, but also costs you more on a per-serving basis. It's much less expensive (and just as effective) to use 100% whey protein powder and add your own carbs to the post-workout snack. See, if you go with the carb-and-protein powder, you have to pay by weight for the product even though carbs aren't nearly as expensive as protein. You'll have to weigh taste, convenience, and cost when selecting your post-workout nutrition. Regular food can work fine in place of protein powder – regular food containing protein takes longer to digest than the powder, but if you eat right after you work out that won't be an issue. In spite of the hype you see from supplement companies, how quickly your post-workout nutrition hits the bloodstream isn't as important as simply following a balanced diet overall. However, if you don't feel like eating after working out, a protein shake is an easy solution. If you'd rather have real food, turn to Reference B for a list of good food choices post-workout.

No matter which option you choose, meal-replacement products and post-workout nutrition products make eating a relatively balanced meal or snack much easier when you are in a rush or out and about. They are usually fortified with vitamins, minerals, fiber, and other beneficial nutrients. Try buying them in bulk to save money.

Even when paying full retail price for a single serving, if you compare meal replacement bars and shakes to the price of convenience store snacks or fast-food, you won't be spending much more grabbing one of these than you would buying junk food.

10. The right way to do fast-food. If you're jonesing for something hot or if you're out with someone who wants to order fast-food, you *do* have options (not a ton, but some) that will allow you to stay on a healthy eating plan. Most fast-food places offer some type of grilled chicken sandwich – you can order this with extra lettuce and tomato along with mustard or light salad dressing. Subs made without cheese or mayonnaise are also usually healthy enough. The next best fast-food sandwich to order is a plain hamburger.

Looking at side orders, a garden salad or chicken salad should be okay, but try to do without added bacon, croutons, or full-fat cheese. Full-fat dressing should be used sparingly, or opt for low-fat if it's offered (stay away from fat-free dressing, since it's usually loaded with sugar). A baked potato without cheese, butter, and sour cream isn't bad as long as you're not following a low-carb plan. Pizza and tacos are okay to have once in a while – just make sure to order a thin-crust pie and ask them to go easy on the cheese for both pizza and tacos.

Even if you order something that's really fattening, the key when dealing with fast-food is to limit yourself to a snack-sized portion and wait until you have access to healthier food to fill up. You don't need to be afraid of fast-food – just be sure to keep the portions down. In Reference B you'll find a more extensive fast-food guide.

I have been preparing my own nutritious food for over ten years and these tips have all worked well for me – they make it much easier to stick to your nutrition plan. When cooking for one, eating healthy can actually be easier and less expensive than eating junk food. Once you set up your system for buying and preparing food, it won't feel like a big deal at all.

People who work Monday through Friday might pick a system such as going grocery shopping on Saturday morning and cooking for the week sometime on Sunday. In this case, you might need to run to the store mid-week for some perishables, but other than that you should be set. You'll be surprised how easy it is to eat healthy once you're in the groove. Good luck!

Reference B. Nutrition Guidelines

Here are some general nutrition guidelines for exercisers. If you follow these guidelines and exercise consistently, you should find yourself losing bodyfat and toning up within no time.

General Nutrition Guidelines:
• If you're going to track calories, use a maintenance figure you know is accurate as a starting point, or see pg. 56 for instructions on estimating your maintenance calories.
• If your primary goal is fat loss, deduct 500 calories from maintenance. If your primary goal is muscle gain, add 250 calories to maintenance. The number you get is your calorie level to shoot for per day.
• If you don't want to count calories, just monitor your weight or the way your clothing fits on a weekly basis and add or take away calories from your current diet according to what has been happening with your body. If you don't want to change your total volume of food, try trading high-calorie items for low-calorie ones or vice-versa.
• Consume at least 1 gram of protein per pound of bodyweight daily.
• Consume 20-30% of your daily calories from fat, and include the equivalent of 3-6 grams of fish oil supplements from essential fatty acids in your diet every day.
• The rest of your daily calories can come from carbs.
• Eat within 1 hour of waking up, and eat 3-6 times a day.
• Include some of each of the 3 macronutrients (protein, carbs and fat) in at as many meals/snacks as possible.
• Consume carbs (1/3 gram per pound of bodyweight) and protein (1/2 as many grams of protein as grams of carbs) with as little fat as possible within an hour after resistance training (the sooner after training the better).
• Drink plenty of water and tea, and particularly green tea.
• Protein shakes made with water or low-fat milk, protein bars, and homemade fresh fruit/vegetable juice might be helpful to supplement your diet.
• Avoid sugar and other refined carbs such as white flour if possible, except immediately after resistance training.
• Use alcohol in moderation or not at all – it can stall weight loss.
• If you struggle to control your calorie intake, avoid caloric beverages in general, since they won't leave you feeling full.

Healthiest sources of protein:
- Turkey (white meat; no skin)
- Chicken (white meat; no skin)
- Seafood (avoid added butter or fried seafood)
- Lean Beef (trim the fat)
    - Lean roast beef
    - Top Round steak
    - Top Sirloin steak
    - 95% lean ground beef
    - Top Loin (strip or New York) steak
- Low-fat Dairy
    - Cheese; reduced fat, mozzarella, feta
    - Milk; skim or 1%
    - Yogurt; fat-free or low-fat
    - Cottage cheese; fat-free or low-fat
    - Eggs; 3 whites to 1 yolk, or 1-2 whole eggs per day
- Whey/Egg/Soy Protein Powder, any flavor

Healthiest sources of complex or fibrous carbs:
- "Old Fashioned" oatmeal
- Other wholegrain cereals
- High-fiber breakfast cereals including bran and Kashi
- Sweet Potato/Yam
- Whole-grain breads
- Peas, beans, and lentils
- Colorful vegetables such as broccoli, carrots, and tomatoes
- Fruits, especially citrus fruits (oranges, grapefruit) and berries

Best sources of the Essential Fatty Acids typically deficient in the U.S. diet:
- Flaxseed and flax oil
- Canola oil
- Walnuts
- Fish (especially cold-water fish) or fish oil capsules
    - Anchovy
    - Chinook salmon
    - Herring
    - Mackerel
    - Albacore tuna
    - Pacific halibut

Other good sources of heart-healthy fats:
- Most nuts, especially almonds and sunflower seeds
- Peanut Butter, preferably with no added sugar
- Olive oil
- Sunflower oil
- Sesame oil

Some Breakfast ideas:
- Higher protein bars such as:
  - MET-Rx Protein Plus
  - Pure Protein
  - Balance bars
  - Any bar with at least 20 grams of protein and less than 10 grams of fat
- Hard-boiled egg or omelet w/ low-fat cheese and veggies
- High-fiber cereal with low-fat milk
- Yogurt or cottage cheese with fruit or cereal
- Fruit and string cheese
- Protein pancakes (use 1 scoop vanilla-flavored protein powder, 1 egg, and 3 egg whites, plus cinnamon if desired. Beat and cook like regular pancakes)
- Protein shake smoothie (use 1 scoop of protein powder, 1 cup of milk, ice and/or a handful of fruit)

Good post-resistance-training) choices:
- Pasta salad w/ small amount of dressing (low-fat dressing is better here) and chicken
- Rice or pasta and chicken
- Pizza, light on the cheese and oil
- Turkey, ham, or roast beef sandwich, sub, or wrap (avoid full-fat cheese and mayonnaise)
- Oatmeal prepared w/ low-fat milk
- Breakfast cereal w/ low-fat milk
- Lean meat, vegetables, and a potato or roll
- MET-Rx Big 100 bar
- Power bar, regular Pria bar (not the low-carb version), Cliff Bar, or Luna Bar if you're on the run, followed by a high-protein meal 2 hours later
- Protein shake plus a high-carb snack such as a small bagel
- Low-fat ice cream or frozen yogurt, plus a protein-containing snack

Supplements with clearly measurable benefits:
(Personal needs must be analyzed on a case-by-case basis)
 –Multivitamin/mineral
 –Antioxidant formula
 –Extra vitamin C and E ("extra" meaning beyond what you'd get in a typical multivitamin/mineral that supplies 100% of the RDA for most nutrients)
 –Extra calcium, magnesium, and zinc
 –Fish oil capsules
 –Flax oil
 –Glucosamine Chondroitin
 –Creatine Monohydrate
 –Glutamine
 –Green tea extract
 –Meal replacement products
 –Protein powder and protein bars

"The 80/20 Rule" and Eating in Moderation

Now that you know which types of foods will help you improve your health, your fitness, and your appearance, should you strive to eat that way all the time? Unless you're planning to model or compete in a bodybuilding or figure show in the next six weeks, the answer is "no." Your body certainly thrives when your diet is composed predominantly of healthy, nutritious foods. However, it usually doesn't make much difference, especially in the long run, if you have "junk" food once in a while. Think of your nutrition in the context of the "80/20 Rule."

To follow this rule, 80% of the time you should choose healthy, nutritious foods, and 20% of the time you should choose "fun" foods for the sake of taste, variety, pleasure, and socializing. Once your body has the nutrients it needs (the 80% part) the rest of your calorie sources don't matter as much. I want to stress that you should *trade* some of your "healthy" meals and snacks in for other items, rather than eat all your healthy meals and snacks *plus* the other stuff (that way your total calorie intake won't be too high). You might end up with a few more calories than usual when you trade the healthy for the not-so-healthy, but that's fine since 80% of the time you'll be eating really clean.

If you follow the 80/20 Rule, you are more likely to be healthy and achieve your goals in the long run than someone who strives for a perfect nutritional regimen all the time. The person who tries to be superstrict is at a high risk for giving it all up, and the benefits to being *that* strict are negligible. Plus, one of the great things about working out is that you can "get away" with eating some junk food without it showing up on your hips because you're burning calories when you exercise. In fact, sometimes people who exercise run the risk of eating too *few* calories, particularly when they try to eat only the healthiest foods. Perhaps the most important argument for the 80/20 Rule is that letting go and enjoying life is part of what constitutes a healthy lifestyle. You should feel free to have the occasional birthday cake, piece of pizza, or beer if you want it. As long as you don't do it all the time, having those treats shouldn't affect your weight loss. In fact, after you indulge you will be more motivated to stick to your diet.

Some people go off their healthy diet plan for a full 24 hours once a week or so – they have a planned "cheat day." Many people find that this works well for them, meaning that they make steady progress towards their goals while incorporating a cheat day every 5-

10 days. In general, though, cheat days work best for those who exercise very hard. I don't feel that they are the best approach for the average person. The reason is that many people will go too far overboard on their cheat day and sabotage their progress, particularly if they don't burn many calories exercising. If you don't exercise vigorously 5-6 days a week, you're probably not going to have as much leeway to indulge. On the other hand, you might try having a weekly cheat day and find that it works very well for you, particularly if you work out at least five days per week and you really push yourself.

For most people, it seems to fit their needs and schedule better to have a couple of "cheat meals" per week rather than one entire cheat day. When you go that route, you can enjoy a couple of social meals or satisfy a couple of cravings without going off your diet plan – the extra calories in those meals shouldn't be enough to stall your weight loss. If your cheat meals *do* seem to stall your weight loss, try cutting down the portion sizes of your cheat meals, but still choose whatever you'd like to have for those two meals per week.

Before I continue on the 80/20 Rule, I'd like to mention plain old portion control. Some people aren't up for a drastic overhaul of their diet and would prefer to diet by cutting back on portion sizes while continuing to eat the foods they're used to. That's a fine approach to dieting, particularly if you just want to get smaller, but not necessarily reach a super-low bodyfat percentage (but rather, end up right in the middle of the healthy range for bodyfat percentage). To practice portion control, as long as you're eating a reasonably nutritious diet you don't need to alter your way of eating much, but you should try to stick to smaller portions of what you're used to eating or what you enjoy most. As long as total calories are kept at an appropriate level and you're exercising, you should be able to shed fat using this approach.

No matter what you decide to do with your diet, treating yourself like a robot by thinking "food as fuel" all the time without ever taking the opportunity to indulge isn't the way to go, especially in the long-term. You will be happier and healthier all around by allowing yourself to be human and allowing yourself to enjoy the journey of losing fat and improving your body.

Now I'm going to discuss what happens when you allow yourself to deviate from your diet plan – and don't worry, because it's a good thing! Besides the psychological benefits of the 80/20 Rule, there are physiological reasons why you should stray from your regular diet from time to time. Remember how I said that rest days and rest weeks are an important part of your workout plan? It isn't to your advantage to go for 100% intensity all the time. Less really can mean more. With diet, people tend to get better results sticking to the 80/20 Rule all the time than they do trying to be "perfect" all the time. This is partly due to adherence issues, since most people simply won't be able to follow a "perfect" diet for a variety of reasons – either they are on the road much of the time, or they go to dinner parties regularly, or they experience such intense food cravings that they can't help but give in. They are more likely to adhere to an 80/20 plan and more likely to quit a plan dictating that they must be "perfect." Also, it's easier to be strict with yourself when you know you can have the other foods sometimes, just not at the moment (this helps to reduce your *urgency*, a concept from Strategy 15)

Believe it or not, though, in some cases people who follow 80/20 actually get leaner than people who literally *are* "perfect" all the time with their diet. Being perfectly strict with dieting doesn't tend to work well in the long run. Your body will eventually catch on and your metabolism will slow down when you follow a strict diet plan day after day. Your body does this to prevent you from losing all your excess bodyfat, since it's not sure if you'll ever go back to eating at your maintenance calorie level. So, a cheat meal or even an entire day off plan "tricks" your body into believing that it doesn't have to worry because there is plenty of food available.

Your body will adapt to any situation it experiences over and over. The reason drastic changes in diet tend to work well in the beginning is because your body takes a little while to "catch on" and switch gears to adapt to what you're eating. This is one reason why cyclic plans for diet usually work well. By following a cyclic diet plan, you get to take advantage of the window of time before your body catches on to the new diet. See, your body is capable of adapting so that it runs mainly on whichever fuel is the most abundant in your body. That's why weight loss always comes down to calories-in versus calories-out, whether you follow low or high-carb, low or high-fat, or anything in between.

However, unless you're really lean already, you don't need to use cyclic dieting to make great progress and avoid adaptation to the dieting. "Cheat" meals here and there will suffice for this purpose for most people. Eating more carbs and more calories once in a while usually results in a boost to metabolism for a few reasons:

1. The actual act of eating and digesting food requires calories, which means that eating is a thermogenic (calorie-burning) activity and you see a bump in BMR when more food is consumed.

2. When your body is confident that food is not scarce, it is less likely to "hoard" energy (as bodyfat).

3. If you eat off your diet plan and then get strict again, your body will usually respond with fat loss. However, if you always eat the same way you will tend to plateau pretty fast. The other thing you must realize is that it is nearly impossible to gain bodyfat from one snack, meal, or even one day of overeating – this is because, particularly if you work out, your muscles can store over a day's worth of glycogen (carbs) before you'll put on a significant amount of bodyfat. As long as you are back on track by the next day or two and you didn't eat all high-fat foods, you won't gain an ounce of bodyfat from one day of overeating. All you'll gain is temporary water weight on the scale, and as a bonus you'll be stronger and more energetic in the gym, which means you'll be able to burn more calories during your workout.

4. Treating yourself once in a while tends to alleviate the urge to ditch your diet completely, which saves calories in the long run.

Give the 80/20 Rule a try – I'm sure you'll be happy with the flexibility and the results!

Artificial Sweeteners

Although I only provide an overview on nutrition in this book, I feel that it is important to cover artificial sweeteners. The one I believe to be the most harmful is aspartame, sold under several trade names including NutraSweet and Equal. Many food and beverage products are made with aspartame, and aspartame is also sold as a table sweetener (the blue packets). Personally, I used to consume aspartame all the time, but I won't touch the stuff anymore. I used to be naïve enough to believe that anything sold in this country wouldn't be an inherently harmful substance. The fact that cigarettes are sold at every street corner seems to make that logic fall apart, but I guess I considered foods and beverages to be different. Even alcohol isn't *all* bad, particularly when consumed in moderation. There are indeed a few health benefits associated with alcohol.

However, consuming aspartame won't improve your health one bit, and the evidence suggests that everyone is harmed by aspartame on some level. People who support aspartame argue that it's better for you than sugar, but who's really to say which is the lesser of two evils? At least sugar isn't composed of potentially toxic chemicals. Anyone who thoroughly researches aspartame would agree that it's one of the most dangerous substances on the market that is added to foods. I realize that this remark may seem to be a bit alarmist, but I say it because I've witnessed firsthand what has happened to several people I care about when they became regular users of aspartame. Miraculously, just weeks after ceasing its use, their symptoms virtually disappeared.

Aspartame accounts for *over 75 percent* of the adverse reactions to food additives reported to the FDA (15). Many of these reactions are very serious, and include seizures and death. Here is a short list of symptoms reported as being caused by aspartame: Headaches/migraines, dizziness, seizures, nausea, numbness, muscle spasms, weight gain, rashes, depression, fatigue, irritability, tachycardia, insomnia, vision problems, hearing loss, heart palpitations, breathing difficulties, anxiety attacks, slurred speech, loss of taste, tinnitus, vertigo, memory loss, muscle atrophy, and joint pain. There are actually 90 different symptoms documented as being caused by aspartame. According to researchers and physicians who study it's adverse effects, the following chronic illnesses can be triggered or worsened by the ingestion of aspartame: Brain tumors, multiple sclerosis, epilepsy, chronic fatigue syndrome, Parkinson's disease, Alzheimer's, mental retardation, lymphoma, birth defects, fibromyalgia, and diabetes (16).

Aspartame is made up of three chemicals: aspartic acid, phenylalanine, and methanol. These substances can all be classified as a chemical poison (17). Side effects from the consumption of these substances can occur immediately as acute reactions, or gradually over a period of use. Even if you feel that you've had no reaction or side effect from using aspartame, with chronic use you are leaving yourself susceptible to the long-term damage that can be caused by the excitatory amino acids found in aspartame. If you have a condition that can't seem to be alleviated by drugs, supplements, or herbs, aspartame consumption could very well be the cause of your problems. For a full list of adverse reactions and side effects, see http://www.holisticmed.com/aspartame/suffer.faq.

I have seen many of my friends and family restore their health by ceasing use of aspartame. I have also experienced symptom relief myself when I stopped using this sweetener. It is amazing to witness the dramatic improvements in health and well being as a result of giving up aspartame. I am horrified that this stuff can be bought by the caseload with no warning label anywhere in sight. At the very least, there should be a warning label regarding the quantity that's "safe" to consume. The original argument given by those supporting aspartame was that people wouldn't be consuming enough of it for a significant effect to occur. If this is the case (and it really acts as a *poison* when consumed in enough quantity) there should at least be a label on products made with aspartame to let people know they can't consume the stuff all day and expect to stay healthy (16). Today, aspartame can be found in a wide variety of products including soda, juice, gum, cookies, cakes, candy, mints, gelatin, pudding, popsicles, and nutrition bars and nutrition shakes of all things.

I suspect that the mounting complaints against products containing aspartame will eventually lead to them being removed from the shelves. Until that time comes, please tell everyone you know about the dangers, and register a complaint with the FDA if you find your health improving after you've stopped using aspartame.

Ironically, despite worries that saccharin might cause cancer (it may cause tumor growth in laboratory animals), saccharin doesn't appear to be nearly as bad for you. Saccharin, used in many food products and sold as a table sweetener under the trade name "Sweet n' Low" (the pink packets) is the sugar substitute that's carried the warning label all these years. I find this very ironic given that there is more evidence aspartame can be detrimental to human health than there ever was for saccharin.

Sucralose is a sweetener that has come into popularity over the past few years – many people who have become fearful of the effects of aspartame are switching to sucralose, sold under the trade name Splenda. It's been used as a sweetener in beverages for several years, and now more and more foods are being sweetened with sucralose – including ice cream and children's breakfast cereals.

Sucralose, although calorie-free, is derived from sugar, and that is the trump card for people who insist that it's "natural" and "harmless." Although you may have heard that it passes through the body undigested, that simply is not true. 20-40% *will* be digested and the toxins can accumulate in your organs (18). There have only been a handful of studies done on sucralose, amounting to less than 1% of the studies that have been done on aspartame and saccharin. There have been no long-term studies at all. I recommend staying away from sucralose and other artificial sweeteners that haven't been studied extensively until we know more, and I definitely wouldn't give sucralose or any other artificial sweetener to kids, because at their lower body weight any potentially harmful substance will do far more damage. At this point, with what we know about artificial sweeteners (which admittedly is not very much in some cases, but it's better to be safe than sorry), aspartame should be your last choice.

A more cautious move would be to avoid artificial sweeteners altogether. If you decide to go this route, you might use sugar in moderation, or consider using a natural alternative to sugar. There are several, but you must develop a taste for them. Stevia, a sweet herb, is the most popular natural alternative to sugar. Some people complain of a slight aftertaste when using Stevia, which may lessen with repeated use. Another alternative sweetener that works well for baking is Gymnema Sylvestre. This herb is particularly useful as an aid in reducing sugar in your diet because it can help reduce sugar cravings, while at the same time serving as a calorie-free sweetener.

If aspartame is so bad for you, why the widespread consumption? Part of the problem is simply ignorance to the dangers, seeing that the company selling it is taking great pains to keep things quiet. However, plenty of people have heard that this sweetener might be harmful. People sometimes turn the other way when they hear that aspartame is harmful because they have been brainwashed into thinking they need aspartame to keep their weight down. It is all too common for people to choose vanity over health (the tanning industry is a good example of this). In spite of the cries that aspartame is a bona-fide poison, people think their low-calorie sweets and drinks are keeping them from ingesting too many calories.

By comparing notes with other fitness, nutrition, and medical professionals, the overweight people we see suffering from problems with their liver and/or metabolism aren't being helped one bit by aspartame. If anything, aspartame puts more unwanted weight on their bodies. There are logical explanations for the fattening and bloating effects of aspartame. When you ingest aspartame it is absorbed from your intestines and then passes immediately to your liver. Your liver then breaks down (metabolizes) aspartame into its toxic components: phenylalanine, aspartic acid, and methanol. This process requires a great deal of energy from your liver, which leaves less energy remaining in the liver cells. When the liver cells have less energy for their functions, which include burning fat for energy, fat burning slows and fat storage increases. Excess fat may build up inside the liver cells causing "fatty liver," and when this starts to occur it becomes extremely difficult to lose weight. Any time your liver is overloaded you'll have a tendency to gain weight easily (19).

Aspartame also can cause weight gain by other mechanisms. It causes an unstable blood sugar level in some people, which increases appetite and sets off cravings for sweets/sugar. Aspartame also causes fluid retention in some people, which gives the body a puffy and bloated appearance. The toxins from aspartame are stored in the fat cells, which can make bodyfat look puffier. The combination of "puffier" fat and water retention makes people appear to have more bodyfat than they really do, and it worsens the appearance of cellulite.

One of the components of aspartame, the amino acid phenylalanine, tends to outcompete all the other amino acids at enzyme sites in the body. When this happens, the formation of dopamine and serotonin is suppressed. As you may be able to guess, it's not a good thing when your serotonin levels are suppressed. Serotonin is the neurotransmitter that reports carbohydrate metabolism. When your serotonin levels are blocked from rising as they normally do when you eat carbohydrates, you wind up craving more and more food even if you're eating enough calories to maintain your weight. The neurotransmitter dopamine is equally as important. Dopamine must be released in order for you to feel satisfied, so when you use aspartame you'll most likely experience insatiable cravings (20). The neuroexcitotoxins present in aspartame also act in the brain to stimulate appetite. This is one of the reasons manufacturers put aspartame and other substances containing neuroexcitotoxins into foods. Even if it doesn't improve the taste of the food, the food will *seem* better tasting to you because your appetite will be stimulated.

Looking at all this information, it's hard to make the case that aspartame is diet-friendly *or* safe! In my opinion, aspartame isn't helpful when you're on a diet, and actually could sabotage your diet. Can you lose weight in spite of your Diet Coke habit? Probably. Will you lose as much or be as healthy if you consume aspartame? Probably not. You are the only one who can decide if the risks are worth it to you. If you're hesitant to give up aspartame, eliminate it from your diet for a one-month trial period to see if you notice a difference in the way you look and feel. During that time, be sure to drink plenty of water to help cleanse your liver and flush the toxins out of your system.

Alcohol

I'll start with the good news – you can definitely indulge in a few drinks here and there and still enjoy steady weight loss and bodyfat reduction, particularly if you exercise. Now, for the not-so-good news: *Drinking has a detrimental effect on your body above and beyond the calories the drinks contain.* Not only does alcohol reduce the number of calories from fat you burn, but it also increases appetite, increases the storage of abdominal fat in particular, and lowers your testosterone level for up to 24 hours after you finish drinking.

According to conventional wisdom, the infamous "beer belly" is caused by excess alcohol calories being stored as fat. Yet, the reality is that less than 5% of the alcohol calories you drink are converted into fat. If this is the case, what's the problem with drinking?

The main effect of alcohol is to reduce the amount of fat your body burns for energy. In fact, after having two shots of vodka, lipid oxidation (the measure of how much fat your body is burning) drops to just 25% of what it would be normally (21)! Although a small portion of alcohol *is* converted directly into fat, your liver converts most of it into a substance called acetate. The acetate is then released into your bloodstream, where it *replaces* fat as a source of fuel.

The combination of alcohol and a high-calorie meal is especially fattening (not that this *ever* happens in real life...) Alcohol increases appetite and decreases inhibitions to overeat, and any food calories you ingest are more likely to be stored as bodyfat if you're drinking at the same time. Even if you manage to stick to your regular diet while drinking, calorie-for-calorie alcohol does more damage to your waistline than any other food.

Drinking alcohol is also one of the fastest ways to slash your testosterone levels. Just a single bout of heavy drinking triggers the secretion of the muscle-wasting and abdominal-fat-storage hormone cortisol and increases the breakdown of testosterone for up to 24 hours. The damaging effects of alcohol on testosterone are exacerbated when you exercise before drinking. What's so bad about a drop in testosterone? To understand, you need to know what effects testosterone has on the body. Testosterone cues the body to increase muscle mass and decrease bodyfat, which means that you have a higher metabolism and have better body tone when your testosterone levels are normal. The increase in testosterone levels is the main reason that teenage boys can put on muscle and drop fat automatically as they grow. The negative effect of alcohol on testosterone levels is one reason that people who drink a lot tend to carry less muscle. It also explains why young men can sometimes drink quite a bit yet remain muscular and lean – in his early 20s a man's testosterone levels are the highest they will ever be – high enough that even heavy drinking won't bottom them out. By the time he's a little older, though, he'll start to notice a significant loss of muscle and a gain in bodyfat if he continues drinking.

While the odd drink now and then isn't going to hurt long-term, the reality is that alcohol and a leaner, stronger body just doesn't mix. Alcohol will also increase the amount of fat around your waistline, even if your overall bodyfat levels aren't very high. If you want to continue drinking on a regular basis (more than three or four drinks a week, spaced out across the week), you'll have to cut back that much more in other areas of your diet, or else work out a bit extra, if you're serious about getting lean. And if you want an elite physique, you will need to give up drinking entirely for a period of time to allow your body to shed the last bit of fat (22).

Drink	Amount (fl oz)	Calories
Beer, light	12	105
Beer, regular	12	145
Bloody Mary	5	116
Daiquiri	2	110
Gin & Tonic	7.5	170
Manhattan	2.5	130
Margarita	3	170
Martini	2.5	155
Pina Colada	4.5	260
Tequila Sunrise	5.5	190
White Russian	3.5	270
Rum (100 proof)	1.5 oz.	125
Vodka (100 proof)	1.5 oz.	125
Whisky (100 proof)	1.5 oz.	125
Brandy (fruit flavored)	1.5	130
Peppermint Schnapps	1.5	125
Burgundy, red	4	95
Burgundy, white	4	90
Champagne, dry	4	105
Port, ruby	4	185
Port, white	4	170
Zinfandel, red	4	90
Zinfandel, white	4	80
Wine spritzer	12	120

Eating Out the Healthy Way

When you're considering what to order at a restaurant, start by reading item descriptions. If they aren't available on the menu, ask your server what's in the meal and how it's prepared. Dishes based on fruits, vegetables, and whole grains tend to be lighter options as long as they aren't drowned in oil. Lean protein sources such as poultry and seafood are also diet-friendly, assuming they're not fried or covered in creamy/oily sauces. You'll want to look for cooking terms that can give you a basic idea of the dish's nutritional makeup. Look for descriptions that indicate low-fat preparation or ingredients because those items will contain fewer calories.

Choose:
–Baked
–Broiled, no added butter
–Grilled
–Poached
–Roasted
–Steamed
–Sautéed w/ broth or little/no oil
–Stir-fried w/ broth or little/no oil

Avoid:
–A la king
–Alfredo, unless low fat
–Au gratin
–Basted
–Breaded
–Buttered
–Roasted
–Creamed
–Fricasseed
–Fried
–Hollandaise
–Sautéed/stir-fried in heavy oil

In most restaurants it is possible to find healthy items within each course of the meal. Here are some pointers for when you're wading through the choices:

Appetizers. Choose appetizers made with fruits, vegetables, or fish. Shrimp cocktail is a great choice. Avoid fried or breaded appetizers.

Soup. Choose broth-based or tomato-based soups such as minestrone, vegetable, or gazpacho. Cream soups, chowders, pureed soups, and fruit soups quite often contain heavy cream or egg yolks. Ask for a list of ingredients to be certain.

Salad. Order lettuce or spinach salad with dressing on the side. Dip your fork into the dressing instead of pouring it onto your salad. Use a full-fat dressing sparingly, or choose a low-fat dressing with no added sugar. Avoid non-fat dressings unless you're sure they don't have added sugar. Caesar, Greek, chef, and taco salads are traditionally high in fat and calories. If you ask for dressing on the side and go easy on (or skip entirely) the cheese, eggs, and meat, these salads will be a lot less fattening.

Bread. Choose whole-grain products if possible. If you are having pasta, skip the bread basket entirely – your meal will contain plenty of carbs. Avoid muffins, garlic bread, and croissants – they're loaded with calories and fat. If you have a bread basket at your table, take one piece and ask your server to remove the basket. Use small amounts of added fat on your bread if you use any at all. You're better off using olive oil instead of butter or margarine.

Side dish. Choose a baked potato, sweet potato, steamed vegetable, or rice instead of french fries, potato chips, onion rings, or mayonnaise-based salads. Ask that the potatoes, vegetables, or rice come without butter or cream sauce.

Entree. Look for descriptions that indicate low-fat preparations, such as London broil, grilled chicken breast, lemon-baked fish, and broiled shish kebab. Avoid items with high-fat descriptions such as prime rib of beef, veal parmigiana, stuffed shrimp, fried chicken, fettuccine alfredo, filet mignon with bearnaise sauce, shrimp tempura, and fried rice. Choose pasta primavera or linguine with red tomato or clam sauce. Skip pasta with meat or cheese stuffing or sauces that contain bacon, butter, cream, or eggs.

Dessert. Finish the main meal before ordering dessert. By the time you're done, you may not even want it. If you do order dessert, split it with your companions or take half home. Tasty and lower-calorie dessert options include fresh fruit, gelatin, angel food cake, sorbet, and sherbet.

You can save fat and calories simply by paying attention to what you're ordering and cutting back on the extras. Many people instinctively add salt, butter, sauces, and dressing to their food – sometimes before they taste it. Well-prepared food needs minimal enhancement. If you choose good restaurants you shouldn't need to add anything to the food. Also, when you add butter and salt your taste buds will come to expect it and you'll lose appreciation for the natural tastes of food. Stay away from the extras for two or three weeks and your taste buds will "wake up" and become more adept at picking up the subtle tastes of food. That means you won't even miss the butter and salt!

If your meal comes with sauce or dressing, ask for it on the side and just dip your fork into it before taking a bite. This allows you to enjoy the sauce while limiting the amount you consume. Also, keep in mind that you can always substitute healthier condiments for what is typically offered. For example, use mustard rather than mayonnaise, or pepper or lemon juice instead of salt.

Also, watch what and how much you drink. Many beverages contain a substantial number of calories. For example, a large soda (32 oz.) has about 400 calories. Alcohol puts a block on fat burning and stimulates the appetite. Instead, order water, seltzer with lemon, or unsweetened iced tea. If you want a hot drink, try coffee or tea, either black or with a little milk. If you can't get used to taking it that way, go easy on the cream and sugar.

Many times the problem with eating in restaurants is not so much the *type* of food, but rather the *quantity* of it. The average restaurant serves oversized portions, which means that your meal will contain too many calories for one sitting. You should keep your portions small even when there is a large amount of food in front of you. When you keep portions small you'll also be able to enjoy a wider variety of foods during the meal, while still keeping total calories under control. This is good for your health because having a variety of foods means getting a variety of nutrients – you'll be sure to get all of the energy, protein, vitamins, minerals, and fiber you need.

Though it may cost more, ordering a la carte will allow you to enjoy a variety of foods in diet-friendly quantities. Try making a meal out of broth-based soup (avoid cream-based soup) along with some appetizers. When ordering the appetizers, be sure to generally select broiled, baked, or steamed appetizers rather than their deep-fried counterparts. Try these other suggestions for keeping your portion sizes down:

1. Ask if you can have a lunch portion, even if you're eating dinner. Or simply request a smaller portion, even if you have to pay the same amount. If you decide to order the entire meal, you might want to request a to-go container when the meal arrives. Immediately put half of the food in the container to have as leftovers the next day. When it's difficult to gauge the portion size of a particular food item on the menu, such as toppings for a baked potato, ask for it on the side. That way you'll be able to control how much you add.

2. Plan to split a meal with a companion, particularly when you know the restaurant serves large portions.

3. Eat only until your hunger is satisfied. If you're tempted to clean your plate, ask your server to remove the dishes.

Buffets may prove especially challenging when you're trying to eat smaller portion sizes. Large amounts of food and the freedom to go back for seconds (or thirds!) can easily lead to excess. It can also be tempting to regard buffet dining as a personal challenge – some people stuff themselves just so they can get their "money's worth." On the other hand, buffets can be ideal when you're trying to eat healthy because you'll have a wide selection to choose from and you can see what you're "ordering." You'll get to take the amounts you want, which is great as long as you exercise some self-control. To limit the amount of food you eat, survey the entire buffet line before you start piling things onto your plate. Then decide what you want and stick to your plan. Start with salad minus the high-fat dressings and toppings, such as cheese and croutons. The salad will start filling you up without adding many calories. Then you can go back for an entree. Fill up on plenty of vegetables that don't have added butter, margarine, or sauces.

Fast-Food on a Diet

Many meal options at fast-food restaurants contain staggering amounts of fat and calories. For example, a meal of a double cheeseburger, large fries, and a medium soda has about 1,500 calories and 65 grams of fat. This is an entire day's worth of calories for a sedentary female, or an active female on a weight-loss diet. There is never an instance when you can justify eating that many calories in one sitting.

Some fast-food places do offer lighter fare such as salads and grilled chicken. But watch out for dressings, sauces, and other condiments that can boost your meal's fat and calorie content. You definitely have to be choosy when patronizing fast-food places. These guidelines can help:

- For breakfast, consider fresh fruit, unsweetened fruit juice, cereal with skim or 1% milk, low-fat yogurt or low-fat cottage cheese and fruit, or eggs with lean ham and low-fat cheese.

- Order smaller portions. For example, get a single small hamburger instead of a double, or a small fries instead of a large. Also limit high-fat, high-calorie burger toppings and condiments, such as bacon, cheese, mayonnaise, sauces and dressings.

- Choose poultry items that aren't fried or breaded, such as broiled or grilled chicken or a sliced turkey sandwich. Or choose a sandwich made with lean meats and veggies and healthy condiments such as mustard. Request sandwiches on whole-wheat bread, low-fat or low-carb tortillas, or pita bread.

- Load your plate with fresh fruits and vegetables if the restaurant has a salad bar. Use full-fat or reduced-fat dressing sparingly. Limit cheese, egg yolks, and croutons.

- Remove any breading from your food and use a napkin to absorb extra oil if you order a fried item.

- Choose a baked potato topped with vegetables, or a whole-grain bagel with the butter, cream cheese, or jelly on the side or not at all.

- Cut back on ketchup, mustard, sauces, and pickles if you need to reduce your sodium intake. Other high-sodium items to watch out for are french fries, chips, ham, sausage, bacon, and cheese.

- Avoid milkshakes and dessert items such as pies and sundaes with syrup. Try fresh fruit or flavored coffee with skim milk. Frozen yogurt or angel food cake will be a little higher in sugar but are relatively low-calorie and low-fat.

As you can see, it's definitely possible to eat healthy when you're away from home. In fact, dining out offers a great opportunity to enjoy a variety of healthy foods without having to go through the work of preparing the food or doing the cleanup yourself. Just don't let large portions, unfamiliar menus, and tempting desserts discourage you from trying to eat healthy.

Reference C. Just How Much Time is Required to Experience the Benefits of Exercise ?

How much time do you need to spend working out to see results? Probably less than you think. If you perform four exercises for two sets each three times per week, you can literally experience significant, noticeable results spending just 30 minutes per week working out.

I know of people who take a 30-minute walk once a week, and that is the only exercise they get all week. Walking is a good form of light cardio, but if these people decided to trade that 30 minutes of time spent walking for 30 minutes performing "Fit with Four," they could lose 10-20 more pounds over the course of a year, assuming they didn't change their diet. How? There are two major mechanisms at work:

1. For a 150-pound person, walking for 30 minutes at 4 m.p.h. (a good clip) burns about 160 calories. Lifting weights for 30 minutes will burn about the same number of calories or a little less (depending on how vigorously it's done), but by lifting weights you will induce a post-workout calorie burn in addition to the calories you burn during the actual workout.

2. Assuming you build five pounds of muscle during the course of a year as a result of weight training (not very hard to do if you're consistent about working out), you'll lose over 9 pounds of fat that year and *over 19 pounds of fat* the next year due to the elevated metabolism from the extra muscle tissue (using the conservative estimate of 35 extra calories burned per day for each pound of added muscle). This is, of course, assuming that you keep eating the same way you were eating before you gained that muscle.

Some people happen to enjoy working out and prefer to spend more than 30 minutes per week exercising. You might not, and that's okay. I assure you that if you take 10 minutes three times a week to do the routine I list on the next page, it will be the greatest return on 30 minutes per week that you have ever experienced. It really will blow your mind. Of course, someone that spends more time will get more benefit. It's just that there is a point of diminishing returns with exercise, so the more you do, the less benefit you get in return for each minute you spend exercising. So, even if you never increase the amount of time you spend on fitness, you will still get over half the benefit that's possible to get from exercise by doing your 30 minutes per week.

When you're only exercising for 30 minutes a week, you *will* get stronger and healthier, but your appearance *won't* change drastically at first, especially if your diet isn't great. However, if you stick to a good diet and follow this routine, you'll definitely notice significant changes in your body. And if you add cardio to the mix, you'll see even more changes and they'll come faster for you. Turn to the next page for the exercises.

Fit with Four

If you aren't willing to spend much time exercising or don't know how to perform many exercises, don't worry – it's amazing what 10 minutes spent on simple exercises can do. I have seen people who haven't exercised for years make good progress just by being consistent and working hard during those 10-minute training sessions. If you perform four exercises for two sets each and do that three times per week, you can experience significant, noticeable results spending just 30 minutes a week working out right at home. This routine can be done in any home using a few inexpensive pieces of equipment. Here is the list of exercises, which I call "Fit with Four":

1. **Compound leg exercise:**
   Squat or Lunge
2. **Compound exercise for chest, triceps, and shoulder:**
   Chest Press or Push-up
3. **Compound exercise for back, biceps, and shoulder:**
   Bent-Over Row
4. **Exercise for abdominals:**
   Basic Crunch and Side Crunch, or Bicycles for abs

When presented with this information, what excuse do you have to put off starting a workout routine? If it seems inconvenient or downright impossible to get to the gym or devote an hour a day to working out, there's no need to worry because that's not necessary to achieve a decent fitness level. Please don't be a black-and-white thinker and decide that if you can't be in the gym every day you don't want to work out at all. If you are wary of committing large chunks of time and money on fitness right now, give this routine a try. Keep reading for instructions on how to perform the exercises and pictures of the correct form.

For all exercises, perform 10 repetitions (reps for short) to start. When that's no problem, increase your reps to 12 or 15 at a time. When you're able to complete 15 reps with correct form, increase the weight or move to the more advanced exercise. As a beginner, each rep should take about 4 seconds: 1-2 seconds to lift and 2-3 to return. That means a 15-rep set should take you approximately 60 seconds to complete. Be sure to time your sets every once in a while to make sure you're working at the correct pace.

1. Compound leg exercise

The **squat** is one of the best leg exercises there is. It targets the hamstrings, quads, hips, and butt. The squat also uses the abs, low back, and calf as stabilizers.

First, you need to learn the proper stance for the squat:
1. Stand upright with your feet about one foot wider than hip-width on each side.
2. Turn your toes out slightly.
3. Tighten your abs and tense your low back, keeping the slight natural arch in your spine. Keep your chin up and your eyes straight forward.
4. Assume the "straight leg" position, which for compound leg exercises means keeping a very slight bend to the knee, as it can be harmful to the joint if you completely lock out your knees while they are in a weight-bearing position.

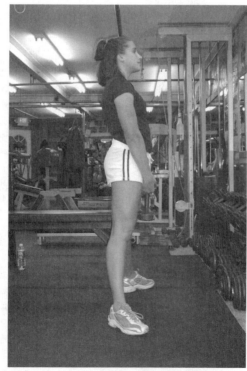

Gina Paolino showing the starting stance for a Dumbbell Squat

Next, you need to learn the proper execution for the squat:
1. Bend your knees until your upper thighs are parallel to the ground. If flexibility or strength limits you, only go as low as you can. Think of sitting *back* into a chair as you bend your knees.
2. Keep your back slightly arched with your butt sticking out a little in the back, and keep your chest up. The motion is similar to sitting down on a chair, with your weight on your heels and your butt shifted back.
3. Keep your shoulders upright and pulled back with your chest slightly out and your eyes straight ahead, and keep your chin up during the exercise. Keep your torso as upright as possible.

At one point, if not now, you will want to add resistance so that this exercise is challenging in the 10-15 rep range. Your options for adding resistance are dumbbells or a barbell.

Dumbbells will be easier to start with and require less equipment:
1. Let a dumbbell hang vertically from your hands by interlacing your fingers around the handle of the dumbbell and pressing your palms against the inside edge of the dumbbell.
2. Let your arms hang straight down and execute the squat.

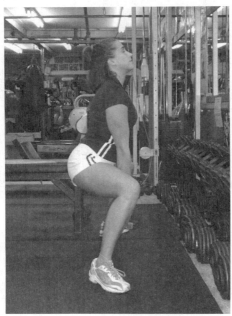

Dumbbell Squat

If you're going to use a barbell, it should be placed across the back of your neck, resting on your upper back and shoulders. If the weight is heavy enough to challenge your legs you will probably need a squat rack, or at least a strong spotter, to help you position the barbell properly and take it on and off your back safely.

1. If you can lift the barbell over your head, lift it up and place it behind your head. If you have a partner, have him place the barbell behind your neck. If you have a squat rack, you should have the pins on the squat rack set a little lower than shoulder height. Duck under the barbell and stand up under it to leave it resting on your upper back.
2. Your hands should be gripping the barbell and should be about 1-2 feet wider than your head on each side (choose the most comfortable position).
3. Execute the squat.

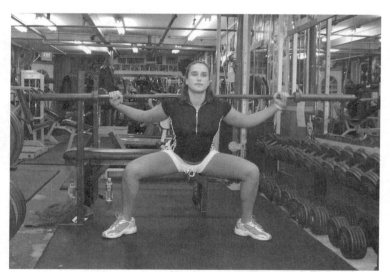

Barbell Squat

Another option for a compound leg exercise is the **lunge**. You might choose the lunge over the squat for a number of reasons:
1. The squat continues to feel awkward even after you've been practicing for weeks, or it causes pain in your knees.
2. You need to use more weight to continue challenging yourself on the squat, but don't have access to it (you can't hold a heavier dumbbell, or you don't have a barbell and a squat rack).

3. You're getting bored with the squat or have been doing it for a while and have reached a plateau.
4. You want more variety in your program.

The technique for walking lunges, the most effective type for general strength training, is as follows:
1. Start by standing fully upright with both feet together.
2. Take a large step forward with one leg, then bend your knees until your back knee is nearly touching the floor. Do not allow your front knee to pass beyond your toes.
3. Keeping your bodyweight on your front foot and leg, press through your front foot to stand. Bring your back leg through and take another giant step forward, this time with the other leg.
4. It's best to have a clearance of at least 8 paces so that you're not turning around constantly – also, keep in mind that, to complete the recommended 10-15 reps for each leg, you will need to do 20-30 steps in total.

Use dumbbells or a barbell when you are ready to add resistance to your lunge:
1. To use dumbbells, simply hold one in each hand.
2. To use a barbell, place it across your upper back.

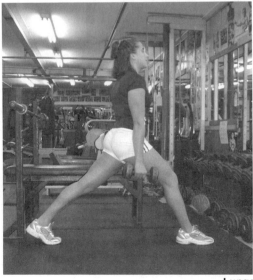

Lunge

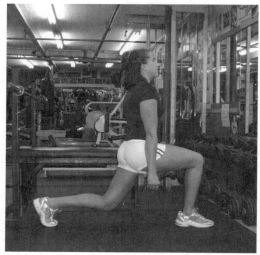
Lunge

2. Compound exercise for chest, triceps, and shoulder

Variations of the **push-up** will target your chest, triceps, and front head of the shoulder. The abdominals, low back, and lateral and rear heads of the shoulder act as stabilizers.

Here is the correct form for the upper body for all variations of the type of push-up you'll do as part of this program:
1. Hands should be about two inches wider than shoulder width, and your nose should be positioned about two inches in front of your fingertips.
2. Your body should remain straight through the hips so that your body forms a straight line (don't allow your butt to stick up).
3. Avoid locking out your elbow, as this can be harmful when there is weight loaded over the joint.

The easiest version is the push-up against a wall. To perform it, stand in front of a wall on your tiptoes with your arms out straight and your palms flat against the wall. Bend your arms until your nose is close to the wall (touch your nose to the wall if you can), then push yourself away from the wall by straightening your arms. Make sure you don't bend your neck forward, but rather maintain a straight neck in alignment with the spine.

If the wall version is easy for you, try a push-up with your hands against a countertop. The higher the countertop is, the easier the push-up will be. Your feet should be positioned so that your chest touches the countertop when you bend your arms. Remember to keep your body straight through the hips, and allow yourself to rise on your tiptoes as you bend your arms during the push-up. Aim your chest to the edge of the countertop, touching it to the edge if you can.

The next higher level of difficulty is a push-up on the floor off your knees. For this version, your hands need to be on the floor with your fingers pointed forward. Bend your knees and cross your feet at the ankles. Be sure to keep a straight body through the hips, meaning that your butt does not stick up. Keep your neck in alignment with the spine and try to touch your nose to the floor.

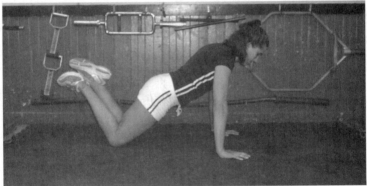

Starting position for the Push-up off the knees

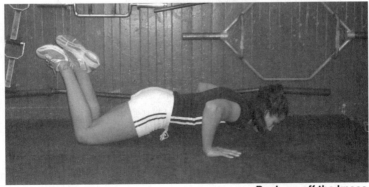

Push-up off the knees

A more advanced option is push-ups on the floor off your toes. If you need something even more difficult so that 10-15 reps challenges you, try weighted push-ups, either wearing a backpack filled with however many pounds you need, or with a friend (or enemy!) pushing on your back.

If you want to change your workout routine at some point, consider dumbbell or barbell chest presses (also called the bench press) in place of push-ups if you have access to the equipment.

For a **chest press** or bench press, you need a flat or incline bench and either two dumbbells or a barbell:
1. Lie on your back on the bench. Start by holding the weights above your chest with your hands 1-2 inches wider than shoulders.
2. If you are using dumbbells, hold them the "long way" so they form one long line.
3. Bend your arms until the barbell is close to or actually touching your chest, or the dumbbells are at the sides of your torso in line with your chest. If you actually touch your chest with the weight you might feel a strain in your shoulders if your flexibility isn't so good. Only go as deep as you can comfortably go.
4. Press the weight back up until your arms are fully extended (if you're using dumbbells, don't *try* to move them in or out while you push – just push straight up by straightening your elbows and the weights will naturally move toward each other a little bit).
5. Avoid locking out your elbows, as this can be harmful when there is weight loaded above the joint.

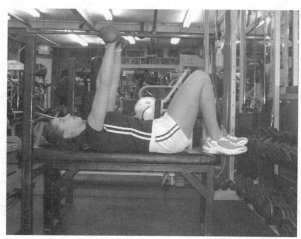

Dumbbell Chest Press

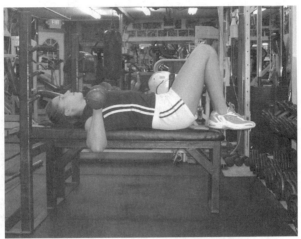
Dumbbell Chest Press

Compound exercise for back, biceps, and shoulder

The **Bent-over row** targets the lats of the back, the biceps, and the rear head of the shoulder. When done standing, bent-over rows also work the low back. The hamstrings, forearms, and quads act as stabilizers during the bent-over row.

The execution is as follows:
1. Start bent-over at the waist with your back at a 45-degree angle to the ground. Bend your knees slightly and arch your back slightly. Stick your butt out a little.
2. Hold dumbbells the "long way" (end to end) or a barbell. With your arms hanging straight down at shoulder width, pull the weights up toward your ribcage by contracting your back muscles (try to squeeze your scapula together). Touch the weights to your abdomen if possible. Elbows will move back beyond the sides of your body, and can be a few inches away from your body.
3. Lower the weights by straightening your elbows until your arms hang straight down from your shoulders.

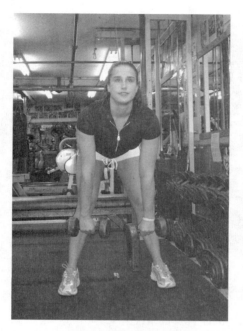
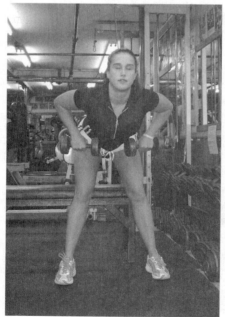

Standing Bent-Over Row

If you find it uncomfortable to stand bent-over as described, you can perform this movement one arm at a time. For the one-arm bent-over row, place one palm on a bench or the edge of a couch. Bend over so that your back is nearly parallel to the ground and hold a dumbbell in your other hand. Hold the dumbbell parallel to your body with your palm facing in toward your body. When you row one dumbbell at a time, you should keep your elbow tucked in close to your body. This version of the exercise (as opposed to the standing one) has its benefits because you'll be able to use a bit more weight and you'll also be able to isolate each lat a little better. However, for a four-exercise routine, the standing version is preferable because it also targets your low back.

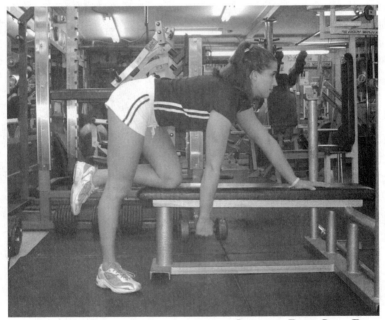

One-arm Bent-Over Row

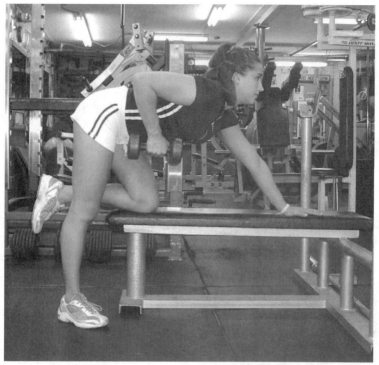
One-arm Bent-Over Row

Exercise for abdominals

The best thing to do for abs when starting a workout routine is the **basic crunch**:
1. Lie on your back on the floor with your knees bent and your feet flat on the floor.
2. Interlace your fingers and place your hands behind your head. Keep your elbows pointing out rather than pulled in close to the ears.
3. Keep your neck straight in alignment with the spine and press your low back into the floor.
4. Contract your abs to lift your shoulders a few inches off the mat.
5. Avoid pulling your neck with your hands (use your hands for support only). Keep your elbows pointed out to the sides.
6. Hold the crunch for a half-second, then lower your body until your upper back touches the mat, but don't touch your head or shoulders to the mat until you are finished with the set. Keep your abs contracted during the entire set.

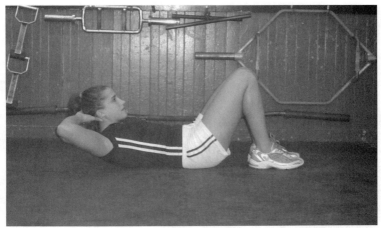

Basic crunch

After you're comfortable with this crunch, you should get acclimated with the **side crunch**. The form is the same for the side crunch, but there are a few variations in the execution. The side crunch targets the obliques and is performed as follows:

1. Lie on your back on the floor with your knees bent and your feet flat on the floor. Lift your left leg and cross your left ankle over your right knee.
2. Once you contract your abs and lift your torso off the floor just like in the basic crunch, start twisting your torso to the left so that your right elbow points toward your left knee. Your elbow should aim toward your knee, but won't come close to touching it if you keep your elbows pointed out to the side like you should. Remember that you don't want to let your shoulders and head touch the floor between reps.
3. Once you've done all your reps for the right side, switch to the left side.

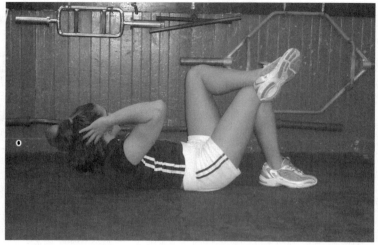

Side crunch

    Bicycles for abs are more advanced. They are tougher and give better results as long as you're ready for them (You're probably ready for them if you can do at least 30 basic crunches and 30 side crunches with no problem). They are also more efficient than most ab exercises because they take care of all the abdominal muscles including the obliques with one exercise. The execution is as follows:

1. Interlace your fingers and place your hands behind your head like you do for the crunch. Lift your shoulders a few inches off the floor by contracting your abs. Legs should be raised slightly off the floor and held out straight. Make sure your low back stays pressed into the floor. If you have difficulty keeping your low back pressed into the floor, hold your legs higher off the ground and bend your knees slightly.
2. Start bending one leg by moving your knee toward your abdomen and twist your torso so that your opposite elbow moves toward your knee. Don't actually try to touch your elbow to your knee – you should keep your elbows pressed out to the sides.
3. Keep scissoring your legs and twisting your torso, and keep shoulders held up off the floor (press your spine into the floor during the exercise and try to curl your back up into a ball). You want the fewest number of vertebrae as possible to remain touching the floor. Keep your legs as low to the ground as you can while keeping your low back pressed into the floor.

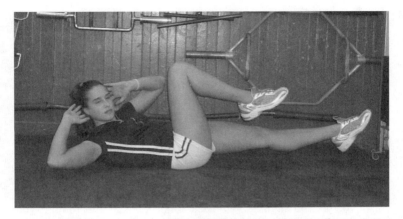

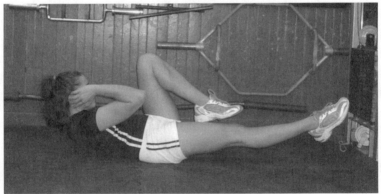

Bicycles for abs

Photo credits:
All photos are of Gina Paolino, courtesy of Bryan Paulhus and Hard Nock's Gym in Amesbury, MA.

"Progressive Resistance Cycle Training"
A systematic, scientific approach to your exercise routine

What I am about to introduce to you is the most efficient fitness program in existence whether you're thinking in terms of time, effort, or money – to follow it, you won't need to work out for an hour or more every day, hire a trainer to watch you work out, or buy expensive equipment or supplements. This program is based on a 6-week "on," 1 or 2-week "off" workout schedule. As long as you're familiar with the basics of a beginner exercise program, you're ready to take the next step, which is to move to an intermediate or advanced workout routine. No matter which type of plan you decide to use, you need to make sure the routine you choose will result in steady progress. You also need to be sure that it has a healthy dose of rest and relaxation built in to allow your body to respond to the work you'll be putting into it.

Muscles grow and fat is stripped away fastest when you "up the ante" with your workouts over time. The number-one reason people stop working out is because they don't feel they are getting the results to justify the time and effort they put into their workouts. That is much less likely to happen when you use progressive resistance techniques.

Progressive resistance techniques can be incorporated into a workout routine with lots of variety if you're experienced in the principles. I am able to offer plans like this to my clients when they see me for training once a week or more. However, if you're not going to use a trainer that frequently, you can still use progressive resistance techniques. Your best bet will be to keep the same exercises during one training cycle of 6-8 weeks to ensure that your progressive resistance is systemized for optimal progress.

Rather than perform a set workout for a period of time and make a change after six weeks or whenever you happen to get bored, Progressive Resistance Cycle Training prescribes the specific weight and number of reps to be used for every workout, and your prescribed weight and/or reps for an exercise will change *every* workout. You will stick to one or two exercises per major muscle group during a given cycle. If you've been through a beginner program, you should already know many of the exercises that will be used because it's the "classics" such as the squat and the bench press that are preferable if you're doing only one or two exercises for each muscle group. The weight and reps to be used for each workout cycle will be planned in advance by your trainer. All you will have to do is follow the schedule and perform what your workout sheet says for the day – no more, no less.

Your workouts will feel easy during the early part of each 2-week cycle and will get harder as the cycle progresses. However, you should be able to complete every workout, even the tougher ones, if your cycle is designed correctly. Not every fitness trainer is familiar with this type of program, but I have studied it extensively and use the principles myself for my workouts. When you use progressive resistance techniques your body will respond to each and every workout, which means that you'll get fair value for the time you put into the process.

Injuries aren't as likely to happen with this type of program because you won't have as many days when you try to push yourself to the limit. And, when you do complete your tougher workouts, because they are strategically placed in the schedule you'll get the maximum benefit for your efforts. Another perk is that even the "easy" workouts will result in progress for you. How?

"Easy" workouts still give you results with this type of program because they are performed when you are coming off a rest week, which means that your body perceives the workout as an increase in stimulus. After all, *anything* feels like a big deal to your body when you're coming off a week or two of rest! Once you grasp this concept, you'll be able to understand the key to this whole program: Every workout results in forward progress because each workout is more difficult than the one before (which your body perceives as "progressive resistance"), but the difference is so marginal that no particular workout will seem that much tougher than the last. Plus, when you get to the harder workouts you'll find that you feel fresh and ready to hit a personal best.

This program makes sense on so many levels, I'm astounded that more gyms and trainers are not spreading the word. I guess many of them don't want to, because they are afraid they might lose you if you are "allowed" to take an entire week or two away from the gym. They also don't want you to see how easy it really is to get in shape, since you'll probably start using their facilities and their products and services less frequently once you realize that you don't have to live in the gym or buy lots of expensive supplements to get in shape.

I don't worry about that because I trust that the results you'll see on this type of program will keep you coming back for more. I'd much rather have a happy client who stays with me in the long-term than a bunch of new clients who pay me tons of money in the beginning, only to quit after a couple of months because they get burned out or are disappointed with their results. I also have faith that you'll spread the word about your great results and I'll be bombarded with referrals. I am so confident my programs work that I stand behind them with my money-back guarantee: Even though you risk nothing by trying them, I have a lot to lose – my entire livelihood and reputation, really – if I don't deliver on what I say.

One of the benefits to you for using Progressive Resistance Cycle Training is that, if you are comfortable with the exercises and form, you'll need to meet with a trainer just once at the end of each 7 or 8-week cycle to evaluate progress and plan your next cycle of workouts. Of course, you may certainly use a trainer more often if you like, and if you choose to do so you'll enjoy the luxury of a top-notch individualized workout based on the same principles behind Progressive Resistance Cycle Training.

Also, keep in mind that these workouts can be completed at home with little or no equipment. This will allow you to save money on gym memberships and/or seeing trainers more frequently.

The weight-training workouts will take 30-40 minutes and are to be completed three times per week. In most cases you'll perform 10-12 exercises for two sets each. You may have cardio in your routine as well, depending on your goals.

Here is an example of a Cycle for one exercise:

Dumbbell Chest Press

Weeks 1 and 2
Workout 1	5 lb x 12 reps
Workout 2	5 lb x 15 reps
Workout 3	10 lb x 12 reps
Workout 4	10 lb x 15 reps
Workout 5	15 lb x 12 reps
Workout 6	15 lb x 15 reps

Weeks 3 and 4
Workout 1	10 lb x 10 reps
Workout 2	10 lb x 12 reps
Workout 3	15 lb x 10 reps
Workout 4	15 lb x 12 reps
Workout 5	20 lb x 10 reps
Workout 6	20 lb x 12 reps

Weeks 5 and 6

Workout 1	15 lb x 8 reps
Workout 2	15 lb x 10 reps
Workout 3	20 lb x 8 reps
Workout 4	20 lb x 10 reps
Workout 5	25 lb x 8 reps
Workout 6	25 lb x 10 reps

Depicted as a chart, Progressive Resistance Cycle Training looks like this:

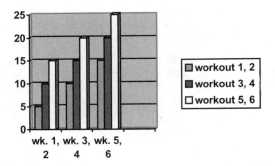

The plans are designed so that your workouts "ramp up" in intensity as you progress through workouts 1-6, which are completed during the first 2-week period. The second 2-week period, weeks 3 and 4, include six more workouts which "ramp up" in intensity just like in the first two weeks. However, this time workout 1 is a bit more intense than it was in the first 2-week period, so you'll end with a workout 6 that is harder than your workout 6 from before. The final two weeks you will once again cycle back and ramp up, finishing at the highest intensity for the entire 6-week period. Then it's time to rest from the weights for a week or two (weeks 7 and 8). You can start the whole process all over again if you'd like to go for another cycle.

You can switch gears to another type of training after one cycle if desired, and should be able to maintain your progress from the cycle as long as you follow a sensible diet and exercise plan. However, most people decide to stick with Progressive Overload Cycle Training for at least for a few cycles. For subsequent cycles, you should try to raise your weights across the board, but only by a small amount. For instance, starting with workout 1, week 1 you'd try 7 pounds instead of the 5 pounds you did during your first cycle for the 12 reps. That means you'd end with workout 6, week 6 at 27 pounds for 10 reps instead of 25 pounds for 10 reps. Relative beginners might be able to increase their weights even more (Keep in mind, brand-new beginners shouldn't use this type of training until they have at least two months of training under their belts).

Most people continue to progress over many cycles if they continue with the training. The rest week sets you up so that even the easy workouts are effective, because your body perceives them as "hard" compared to the past week(s) of rest. Only with this "up-the-ante" system can you make significant progress when you're exercising at less than your maximum capacity. And when you can get the same results using less than your maximum resistance much of the time, you're less likely to get injured or burned out.

Your training regimen might include cardio as well, depending on your goals. If you do cardio, it will be in addition to the resistance-training workouts. You might do your cardio right after resistance training, at another time of day, or on "off" days from resistance training. Just avoid doing cardio anytime in the three-hour window prior to your resistance training.

I have seen people lose weight and bodyfat on this program without doing any cardio at all as long as they're watching their diet. However, you might want to do some cardio to accelerate fat loss if losing bodyfat is your primary goal.

This program is one of the best out there, whether you want to gain muscle or lose fat. The difference between the nature of your results from this program will depend on your calorie intake and on how much cardio you do. A dieter will need to eat sub-maintenance calories (run a calorie deficit) and will need to perform cardio in most cases. Progressive resistance techniques gives dieters the greatest chance to lose fat as quickly as possible while maintaining most, if not all, of their lean body mass. And, as you know, maintaining lean body mass is the key to long-term weight management and permanent fat loss.

A person trying to add muscle will need to eat above-maintenance calories (run a calorie surplus) and generally should avoid cardio. For the person looking to build muscle, progressive resistance techniques result in an ideal anabolic response, assuming that calorie intake is sufficient. When you're "anabolic" and you're weight training, you'll have a favorable hormonal milieu for building muscle. This means that the extra calories you're taking in (the calorie surplus) will go primarily towards muscle growth. This limits the fat gain that tends to go hand-in-hand with building muscle quickly.

Resistance training using progressive resistance techniques is scientifically proven to yield significant results quicker than you'd see with a traditional program, and with minimal risk of injury (12). If for some reason you aren't able to complete the assigned number the reps with good form, it's okay to stop before you've completed the designated number of reps. However, this shouldn't happen under normal circumstances because your trainer will test you beforehand to find the weights and reps that are appropriate for you. This program isn't designed to push you beyond what you are capable of – you actually will have more "easy" days on this program than you would on a traditional program. The funny thing is that you will get better results than you would on a traditional program because you will experience a rebound in strength when you allow your muscles to rest and then ease slowly into working with heavier weights. The pattern of rest followed by a progressive buildup tends to result in an increase in strength when the time comes for the tougher workouts. Quite often people surpass what they *thought* would be the most reps they could get with a given weight because they actually get stronger during the cycle as a result of the systemized training.

Progressive Resistance Cycle Training is the one training method where intermediate and advanced exercisers can gain strength even while they lose bodyweight. This is due to the improved neurological conditioning and the controlled volume of workouts, as well as the strong stimulus for hypertrophy (muscle-building) you get as a result of the systematic increase in resistance. In many cases this program actually allows intermediate and advanced exercisers to "break the rules" and build muscle or at least maintain it while they lose weight.

If you have mastered the form for the basic exercises and have been doing a resistance-training routine for at least two months, you are ready to try Progressive Resistance Cycle Training. The only other requirement is that you can commit to six weeks of three resistance-training sessions a week. It's preferable that you use the same equipment during your cycle. You'll need to know or have tested your maximum weight with varying rep ranges for each of the exercises you'll be using. Your program will be designed according to your individual needs and goals. If you're interested in setting up a progressive resistance plan, please contact me. My contact information can be found near the back of this book.

Reference D. Body Types and Training Suggestions

Before I discuss body types, I would like to present a general guideline for achieving the highest level of fitness and the looks that go along with it.

Please be aware that this program is just a theoretical ideal presented as a tool so that I have something optimal from which I can base personal recommendations. I don't expect nor recommend that you attempt to follow it unless you have a specific reason why you need to be in such extremely good shape.

The reason I say this is, if you take a couple of hours a day on your fitness, you will have to sacrifice in other areas of your life because you won't have time for everything. For the average person, I recommend doing just a fraction of this amount of exercise. It will take you a little longer to get to your goals if you spend less time on exercise, but you will get much more benefit for the amount of time you do spend. In other words, you'll spend much less time exercising, but still enjoy good results. For example, the person who spends about 5 hours a week on fitness will get approximately 90% of the benefit that the person who spends 10 hours gets. It might seem crazy that it takes double the time just to get that last 10%, but you must realize it's that last 10% that sets the elite athletes apart from everyone else. I only show you the "Ultimate Program" so that you understand what's necessary for superior or "elite" results. We are going to take a look at what's optimal and take a look at what you're doing now, and try to land somewhere in the middle. You need to decide what you *can* do and what you *aren't willing or don't have a desire* to do, and go from there.

This program is designed to maximize results for the "natural" exerciser ("natural" meaning you're not taking supplements such as steroids or andro). If you do more than what I have listed in this table, the detrimental effects of overtraining usually start to outweigh any additional benefit you'd gain from doing that much exercise. If you do any less than what you see in these tables, realize that you *are* leaving some results on the table, although your results should still be good and will probably be acceptable to you. This program will need to be modified according to the time and effort you're willing to spend, your goals, and your body type. It assumes that you want a lean, toned look with some visible muscle shape, and that you don't want to be big or bulky.

General Optimal Fitness Plan:

Component	% of total fitness	Prescription for Elite-level Fitness
Resistance Training	40%	4-5 workouts per week, 45-60 minutes each. Use moderate to high-intensity with varying amounts rest between sets. Use any of the classic splits such as a 3-way or a push/pull. Generally work in the 6-12-rep range. Mix up the type of workout by including supersets and compound sets at times, and use circuit training occasionally.
Cardio/Speed Work	30%	4-5 workouts per week. 1-2 workouts moderate-pace 30-45 minutes, 1 workout sprints 20-30 minutes, 1 workout easy to moderate-pace 60 minutes, 1 workout fast-pace 20-30 minutes.
Diet and Supplements	+/- 20%	Can add or subtract from your total. Will vary widely depending on your goals; see "The 7 Keys to Raising your Metabolism for Life" and Reference B for help.
Stress (mental and physical), Sleep and Rest	+/- 10%	Can add or subtract from your total. Includes stress from work, home, and all other mental and emotional stress. Also includes proper amounts of sleep, enough time off from working out, and enough rest weeks per year.

Body Types

We all have inherited specific body types, known as somatypes. There are three basic somatypes: ectomorph, mesomorph, and endomorph. Most people exhibit a predominance of one body type, but also display aspects of the other two (23). Each body type has specific characteristics that have important implications for the design of a fitness program. Genetics play the leading role in determining your body type, and you can only alter your genetic body type so much. Still, you want to make sure you do the best you can with what you have.

To understand why you might have different results from a friend who is using the same program, you must realize that body type dictates basic metabolism and the genetic predisposition toward gaining fat, gaining muscle, losing fat, and losing muscle. Genetically lean people are either going to stay thin no matter what they do, or else find they are able to put on muscle with little or no fat gain as long as they work hard in the gym and start eating more. If you're *not* a genetically lean person, you'll find that you must accept a fat gain along with a muscle gain and that you maintain a relatively high amount of bodyfat even when you're not very muscular.

All of us are programmed by birth to look a certain way. Genetics determine how likely you are to gain weight, and also *where* and *how* you are likely to gain it. Quite often genetically lean people eat more calories than genetically heavy people, but still don't gain weight because they naturally have a faster metabolism. The calorie deficit and calorie surplus rules still hold true – it's just that people have varying responses to overfeeding and underfeeding. Some people start burning more calories to compensate when they eat more, and others don't. Also, some people gain equal amounts of muscle and fat when they gain weight, and lose equal amounts of muscle and fat when they lose weight (they become a bigger or smaller version of what they already were). Others always seem to gain predominantly muscle when they gain weight, and lose predominantly fat when they lose weight. Genetics is the reason you might find that any extra bodyfat you carry appears around your middle or on your hips and thighs. Exercise is the best chance you have to influence the way your body looks in spite of your genetic predisposition.

All this means that people with different body types, and therefore different metabolic rates and body proportions, need to work out a little differently for best results. And, if you have a tendency to gain weight easily, you will need to do more exercise to reach your ideal weight than someone who has a hard time gaining weight. The reason is that you'll need to burn as many calories as you can, whereas people who have a hard time gaining weight will sabotage their efforts in the gym if they burn too many calories.

Endomorphs are heavy-boned as a general rule and have a relatively slow metabolism. Endomorphs tend to store bodyfat easily. Their arms and legs are usually short compared to their torso. Male endomorphs tend to be apple-shaped, storing most of their excess weight in the abdomen. Female endomorphs may be pear-shaped (carrying most of their excess weight in the lower body), apple-shaped, or shaped like an hourglass with a small waist. Their breasts also tend to be larger than average. Endomorphs always seem to be battling with their weight.

Resistance training with little rest between sets along with lots of aerobic exercise will help the endomorph burn more calories. A good amount of cardiovascular work is usually necessary for the endomorph to lose significant amounts of weight. While cardio is essential for endomorphs, they still need resistance training to build muscle. This will increase their BMR so they can burn more calories at rest and during exercise. Endomorphs get the best results with slightly higher repetitions (12-15) during weight training. Besides the positive effect on BMR, resistance training also makes endomorphs smaller, since muscle is denser than fat. Endomorphs need the most exercise of all the body types to reach an ideal weight and get in great shape.

Modified Optimal Fitness Plan for Endomorphs:

Component	% of total fitness	Prescription for High-Level Fitness
Resistance Training	35%	4 workouts per week, 45-60 minutes each. Keep most of the workouts circuit-style, or use supersets (exercises that use opposing muscle groups performed back-to-back) and compound sets (two sets for the same muscle group performed back-to-back). Generally keep reps 12-15.
Cardio/Speed Work	35%	5-6 workouts per week. 2 workouts moderate-pace 30-45 minutes, 1 workout sprints 20-30 minutes, 2 workouts easy to moderate-pace 60 minutes, 1 workout fast-pace 20-30 minutes.
Diet and Supplements	+ 20 or -30%	Can add or subtract from your total. Will vary widely depending on your goals. See "The 7 Keys to Raising Metabolism for Life" and Reference B for help. Pay special attention to keeping calories down. Lower-carb usually works best.
Stress (mental and physical), Sleep and Rest	+/- 10%	Can add or subtract from your total. Includes stress from work, home, and all other mental and emotional stress. Also includes proper amounts of sleep, enough time off from working out, and enough rest weeks per year.

Mesomorphs tend to have square, sturdy bodies and usually are fairly big-boned. Their legs are typically about the same length as their torso. They are athletically built and can build muscle much faster than most people. They are able to lose fat rapidly when on the right diet. Actors Tom Cruise and Arnold Schwarzenegger are examples of mesomorphic body types. If mesomorphs do gain weight, it is generally centered in the abdomen.

Overweight mesomorphs become "apple-shaped," carrying their extra weight around the midsection. Their physique problems when overweight are big bellies and "love handles" on the sides of their torsos.

Mesomorphs generally need a balanced fitness program that includes cardiovascular exercise and a varied resistance-training program. They do best with a mix of high and low-rep work and varying amounts of rest between sets. Turn to the next page for the modified optimal fitness plan for mesomorphs.

Modified Optimal Fitness Plan for Mesomorphs:

Component	% of total fitness	Prescription for High-Level Fitness
Resistance Training	40%	4-5 workouts per week, about 45 minutes each. Use moderate to high-intensity with varying amounts of rest between sets. Use any of the classic splits such as a 3-way or a push/pull. Generally work in the 6-12-rep range. Mix up the type of workout by including supersets and compound sets at times, and use circuit training occasionally.
Cardio/Speed Work	30%	4-5 workouts per week. 2 workouts moderate-pace 30-45 minutes, 1 workout sprints 20-30 minutes, 1 workout easy to moderate-pace 60 minutes, 1 workout fast-pace 20-30 minutes.
Diet and Supplements	+/- 20%	Can add or subtract from your total. Will vary widely depending on your goals. See "The 7 Keys to Raising Metabolism for Life" and Reference B for help. Moderate protein/carb/fat usually works best.
Stress (mental and physical), Sleep and Rest	+/- 10%	Can add or subtract from your total. Includes stress from work, home, and all other mental and emotional stress. Also includes proper amounts of sleep, enough time off from working out, and enough rest weeks per year.

Ectomorphs are typically lean and long-limbed. Most ectomorphs are tall. They tend to have slim hips and small bones in proportion to their height. Ectomorphs generally have a high metabolic rate, making it difficult for them to gain either muscle or fat. If ectomorphs do gain weight, it is usually evenly distributed over the entire body. As ectomorphs age they can develop a potbelly if they don't exercise. Models tend to have an ectomorphic body type. True ectomorphs can perform heavy resistance training and purposefully overeat and still fail to gain significant amounts of weight.

Ectomorphs generally needs less cardio than most and should perform resistance-training exercises using as much weight as they can handle.

If ectomorphs wish to gain size, they should cut back or eliminate cardio, increase their food intake, and focus on weight training.

Modified Optimal Fitness Plan for Ectomorphs:

Component	% of total fitness	Prescription for High-Level Fitness
Resistance Training	55%	4-5 workouts per week, 30-45 minutes each. During most workouts, rest 2 minutes between sets and generally train with 6-12 reps. Train all muscles in the 3-6 rep range at least once per week.
Cardio/Speed Work	15%	3-4 workouts per week. 2 workouts moderate-pace 20-30 minutes, 1 workout sprints 20-30 minutes, 1 workout fast-pace 20-30 minutes.
Diet and Supplements	+ 20% or − 10%	Can add or subtract from your total. Will vary widely depending on your goals. See "7 Keys to Raising Metabolism for Life" and Reference B for help. Keep an eye on total calorie intake to make sure it is sufficient.
Stress (mental and physical), Sleep and Rest	+/- 10%	Can add or subtract from your total. Includes stress from work, home, and all other mental and emotional stress. Also includes proper amounts of sleep, enough time off from working out, and enough rest weeks per year.

Before you jump to conclusions about which body type you have, you must consider the fact that body type and body shape are two different things. All three body types come in four basic body shapes: the cone, the spoon, the ruler, and the hourglass.

The **cone** has wider shoulders than hips. This shape is more common in males and is an "athletic" shape. The **spoon** has narrower shoulders than hips and is typically found in females. The **ruler** is straight up-and-down. In the ruler, shoulders and hips are proportioned and there is hardly an indentation for the waist. The **hourglass** is strictly a female shape. In the hourglass, shoulders and hips have the same measurement but there is a dramatic indentation at the waistline. Keep in mind that excess weight can skew the shape of your body. If you're overweight, look at pictures of yourself at close to your ideal weight to see what your true shape is.

You *can* alter your genetic shape to a point with exercise. One way to do this is by building muscle in certain areas, which will help change your proportions. Building muscle in one area will make other areas look smaller in comparison. For instance, if you build up your shoulders and back, your waist will appear smaller in comparison. While resistance training helps you change the shape of your body, cardio doesn't always do the same. People who do cardio but don't do resistance training tend to simply become a smaller version of what they looked like before. That's because people who do only cardio tend to stay at roughly the same bodyfat percentage – they usually lose both muscle and fat when they lose weight. However, when you do cardio along with resistance training, your body can change dramatically. This is due to decreased bodyfat levels and the aesthetically pleasing shape of the new muscle on your body.

Do not make the mistake of thinking of these somatypes as distinct groups with no overlap. Most people are a blend of 2 or 3 somatypes, but will still exhibit one predominant type. No matter which body type you have, you can't go wrong starting with the general recommendation of 2-3 resistance-training workouts and 2-3 cardio sessions per week. This amount of exercise will give you at least 50% of the fitness benefit you'd get from following the high-level programs. All the extra work you see in the tables is what it takes to get to that top level so few will reach, partly because there are only 24 hours in a day and most of us have a lot of other things going on in our lives that are of more interest or importance to use than changing our bodies that drastically. Also, some people are simply more driven than others to achieve at a high level, and even then we all have different priorities for where we want to direct the majority of our efforts. But no need to worry – you'll still get all the health benefits and many of the appearance benefits from exercise when you bypass the optimal programs and do 2-3 weight-training and cardio workouts per week.

If you choose your plan based on your body type and then cater it to your expectations and goals, you can maximize the benefit you'll get in return for your efforts. Also, if you're familiar with the body types, you'll have more realistic expectations for what you can and cannot change about your body. Everyone can improve her body, but nobody will ever look exactly like someone who has a different body type, no matter what workout she performs or what she does or doesn't eat. There's no need to get discouraged, though, because working out and watching your diet will never fail to get you in great shape and help you make the most of what you have. Also, keep in mind that those who don't have your body type often long for certain features you have that they don't. For instance, a tall, willowy ectomorphic woman might long to have full breasts like an endomorphic woman. Meanwhile, the short, heavier endomorph wishes she had the long, slender legs of the ectomorph. On the male side, the lean and slender ectomorph might wish for the thick muscles of the mesomorph, while the mesomorph longs for the washboard abs that the ectomorph maintains without dieting. The lesson here is to appreciate what you have and learn to let go of what you cannot change.

Reference E. Sources of Information on Diet and Training

I recommend the following books as relatively bias-and-agenda-free sources of fitness information:

–Beyond Brawn by Stuart McRobert
–BodyBuilding 101: Everything You Need to Know to Get the Body You Want by Robert Wolff, Ph.D

These books have exercises and workout routines that can be used as part of a muscle-building or fat-loss program.

In the periodical department, I recommend the following:

–Robert Kennedy's Oxygen Women's Fitness
–Men's Fitness and Health
–Home Bodies monthly newsletter
(had to throw in that plug...)

There are also some excellent websites that can help you design programs and increase your fitness and nutrition knowledge. For your convenience, all of these links can be found on my website, http://www.homeexercisecoach.com. In case you'd like to go directly to them, here are a few websites that I recommend:

–http://www.stumptuous.com/weights.html
This one is written for women, but it's the best beginner fitness and nutrition site that I've seen, and the advice is applicable to both genders.

–http://www.fitnessonline.com
Good for general health and fitness info.

–http://www.intense-workout.com/map.html
Good for diet and exercise plans specifically geared to the goal of adding muscle or losing fat.

http://www.bodyrecomposition.com
This site is for the advanced exerciser who doesn't mind a technical/science bent (it's still written in everyday language) and is interested in training and nutrition theory, cyclic dieting, and the integration of training and nutrition. I use this site all the time to get ideas for my own diet and workouts. The author Lyle McDonald is as knowledgeable as they come.

In addition, I hope you will consider me to be your ultimate resource for all the fitness information you could ever need. My phone and email are always opened to my readers, customers, and clients. All the links I've recommended can be found on my website, www.homeexercisecoach.com. I will be adding links and valuable content to my site as often as I can, making it a great fitness resource for you with all the content fully screened and endorsed by me. You can also subscribe to my newsletter, purchase a select assortment of supplements I recommend, and purchase additional copies of my book on my website.

Home Bodies in-home fitness training
Serving Massachusetts and New Hampshire
    Office Phone: 978-388-3528
    Cell phone: 508-633-7749
    Email: gina@homeexercisecoach.com
    Website: http://www.homeexercisecoach.com

I look forward to hearing from all of you! Call, email, or visit my website to sign up for my monthly Newsletter free of charge. Be sure to take advantage of the coupons in the front of this book, or pass them along to someone who will. And remember, all of my services are fully guaranteed. Just call or email me to schedule an appointment. I'd love to meet you!

Notes

(1) "Beginning Strength Training." <u>UMHS M-Fit Health Promotion Division</u>. April 2004.
<http://www.med.umich.edu/1libr/aha/umfit07.htm>
(2) <u>Robert Kennedy's Oxygen Women's Fitness</u>. Sept. 2004: 18.
(3) Osteoporosis Prevention, Diagnosis, and Therapy. National Institutes of Health, Consensus Development Conference Statement. March 27-29, 2000.
(4) Easton, John. "Lack of sleep alters hormones, metabolism." <u>The University of Chicago Chronicle</u>. 2 Dec. 1999.
(5) Meyer, Paul J. "S.M.A.R.T. Goals." <u>Attitude Is Everything</u>.
<http://www.topachievement.com/smart.html>
(6) <u>Women's Health Weekly</u>. 25 Mar. 2004.
(7) Robbins, Anthony. "Use Quality Qualifiers to Change Your Life" <u>PowerTalk Audio Magazine</u>. 1993.
(8) Sandy Smith. "New Study Links Physical Fitness to Work Performance." March 19, 2004.
<http://www.occupationalhazards.com>
(9) "Appetite suppressants." <u>Cleveland Clinic Health System</u>
<http://diet.webmd.com/content/article/46/2731_1668>
(10) "Andro Side Effects." <www.bodybuildingforyou.com/pro-hormones/andro-side-effects.htm>
(11) Davis, Jeanie Lerche. "Teen Girls' Physical Activity Can Help Prevent Osteoporosis Later On." <u>WebMD Medical News</u>. 11 June 11 2004. <http://my.webmd.com/content/article/88/100005.htm>
(12) McDonag, MJ, Davies CT. (1984) Adaptive response of mammalian skeletal muscle to exercise with high loads. Eur J Appl Physiol. 52(2): 139-155.
(13) Cluett, Jonathan. "Should you ice or heat an injury?"
<http://orthopedics.about.com/cs/sportsmedicine/a/iceorheat.htm>
(14) "10 Tips for Better Sleep." Better Sleep Council.
< http://www.bettersleep.org>
(15) Mercola, Joseph. "Aspartame: What You Don't Know Can Hurt You."
<http://www.mercola.com/article/aspartame/dangers.htm>
(16) "Reported Aspartame Toxicity Effects."
<http://www.holisticmed.com/aspartame/suffer.faq>
(17) Hull, Janet Star. "Aspartame Dangers Revealed."
<http://www.sweetpoison.com>
(18) Mercola, Joseph. "The Potential Dangers of Sucralose." 23 Aug. 2003.

< http://www.mercola.com/fcgi/pf/2003/aug/23/splenda.htm >
(19) Cabot, Sandra. "Aspartame May Cause Weight Gain."
<http://suewidemark.netfirms.com/aspartam.htm>
(20) Carlson, Neil R. Physiology of Behavior. Allyn and Bacon, 2001: 114-120.
(21) Taibbi, R. (1994) "How alcohol affects you." Current Health, 2, 16-19.
(22) <http://www.annecollins.com/calories>
(23) Carson-Cleary. "What's your body type: Endo, ecto or meso?" 20 May 2004. Anchorage Daily.

Index

abdominals, abs 190, 206, 233, 259, 291-292, 296, 303, 305, 320
accountability 82, 102, 104, 116, 120, 129, 139
advanced exerciser 20, 41-42, 44-46, 65, 124, 137, 173-174, 188, 203, 206, 212, 218, 221-222, 243, 291, 298, 305-306, 311, 321
aerobic (*see also* cardio), 124, 158-160, 174-175, 212, 215, 223-224, 315
aerobics classes 49, 132
alcohol 44, 256, 268, 276, 281-282, 324
anabolic 206, 310
anaerobic 159, 181, 212, 215, 223-224
andro 158, 197-198, 213, 233, 312, 323
appetite, 31, 33, 46, 73, 195-196, 213, 221, 225, 254, 279-281, 285
appetite control 46
appetite suppressants 195-196
artificial sweeteners, 276, 278
aspartame 276-280, 323
basal metabolic rate (BMR) 28, 180, 223, 275, 315
basics 136-137, 141, 188, 306
beginner exerciser 36, 41, 45, 137, 141, 149, 173, 183, 201, 205, 223, 233, 235, 254, 291, 306, 310, 321
Bent-over rows 300
binge 33

bioimpedance 162
blockers 195-196
blood sugar 22-23, 46, 279
body composition 47, 155, 202, 221
body shapes 314, 318
body type 114, 117, 161, 210, 229, 312-314, 317-319, 324
bodybuilders 195, 197, 212-213, 233
bodyfat 25, 28-32, 34, 36-39, 41-47, 49, 51-57, 59-60, 63-64, 71, 81, 95-96, 98, 108-109, 120, 139, 159, 161-162, 179, 182, 194-195, 202, 205-207, 209-210, 214-216, 220, 224-227, 268, 273-275, 279, 281-282, 314, 319
bodyfat calipers 108
bodyfat percentage 37, 63-64, 108-109, 139, 161-162, 196, 207, 268, 273, 319
bodyfat-measuring scales 108
breakfast 22, 36, 43, 89, 269, 278, 287
caffeine 65, 193
calcium 64
calorie deficit 24, 27-32, 33, 35-37, 39, 43, 45, 47, 67, 182-183, 194, 206, 216, 222, 224-225, 243, 310, 314
calorie surplus 37, 42, 45, 206, 243, 310, 314
carbohydrate, carbs 23, 29, 47, 57, 181, 215, 279
cardio, cardiovascular

325

exercise (*see also* aerobic) 26, 28, 30-31, 39-40, 46-47, 49, 62, 77, 91, 93, 96, 100, 116-117, 120, 124, 132, 147, 149-151, 158-161, 166, 174, 178-183, 190, 201, 203, 207-209, 212-216, 220-227, 229, 233-236, 238, 243-244, 246, 248, 254-255, 257, 265, 289-290, 308, 310, 315, 318-319
central nervous system 196, 201-202, 253
certified personal trainer, CPT (*see* fitness trainer)
cheat day 272-273
cheat meals 273
chest press, 51, 174, 238, 298
circuit training 178, 183, 234
commitment 11, 15-19, 69-70, 77-78, 84, 128, 175
complex carbs 42, 100, 264
compound sets 234, 313, 315, 317
concentration 151
confidence 14, 17, 33, 88, 91, 102, 106, 163
consistency 83-84, 108, 162, 173
consulting 3, 14, 139, 199
continuous training 126, 139
convenience 124, 131, 263, 266
cortisol 65, 202, 281
cravings, 31, 46, 155, 164, 166, 195, 273, 278-279
creatine, 63, 109, 197
crunch (ab crunch), 175, 303, 305

cutting (fat-loss) 24, 32, 202, 243-244, 273, 284
cycle (training) 45, 117, 206, 236, 243-244, 306-309, 311
cyclic diet 42, 44
diet 14, 23-26, 29, 31-34, 36-37, 39-40, 42, 44-48, 62-63, 65-66, 71, 73-75, 78, 85, 96, 109, 114, 119-121, 123, 127-128, 131, 136-137, 141, 147, 154-156, 164, 178, 182-183, 185, 194-197, 206, 210, 213-214, 216, 224, 243-244, 246, 256, 265, 268-269, 272-275, 278, 280-283, 285, 287, 289-290, 309-310, 316, 320-323
diet pills 194-195
discipline 11, 94, 97, 165, 206, 241
dopamine 279
drinking (*see* alcohol)
drop sets 233
ectomorphs 317-318
essential fatty acids (EFAs) 55, 57, 63, 264, 268
endomorphs, 314-315
endorphins 62, 175
endurance, 158-160, 162, 179, 181, 209, 213, 221, 223, 228, 265
energy balance, 23, 28, 31, 37, 40, 43-45, 195
energy crisis, 32, 38, 66
energy level, 22, 35, 124, 220-221, 242-243, 245
environment, 14, 18, 73, 75, 99, 128, 165, 256
ephedra 193-195
excuse 70, 84, 128, 178, 234, 291
failure (*see* muscular failure)

fast-food 74-75, 186, 267, 287
fat loss 23, 27, 29-32, 34-38, 45-46, 49, 62, 64, 135, 159, 161, 181, 194, 205, 213, 221-224, 233, 236, 265, 268, 275, 310, 321
fat storage 23, 279
fat-burner 193
females 25, 28, 30, 53, 64, 136-137, 146, 180, 182, 197-198, 208, 213-216, 318, 320-321
fiber 57, 154, 196, 264, 266, 269-270, 285
fitness trainer, 14, 60, 82, 95, 97-98, 104, 113-114, 116, 119, 125-128, 131-132, 138-141, 149, 161, 176, 189, 192, 203, 221, 229, 235-236, 242, 246, 250, 306-308, 311
flexibility 120, 140, 248-249, 251, 293, 298
forced reps 150-151, 212, 234
form 12, 15, 41, 44, 64, 95, 100, 139, 142, 149, 173, 187-189, 192, 196-197, 201, 208, 212, 236, 239, 245, 289, 291, 296, 298, 304, 308, 311
fuel (for exercise) 22, 34, 38-39, 42, 44, 46-48, 159, 181, 201, 215, 224-227, 273-274, 281
full-body 51-52, 97, 100, 141, 202, 220, 233
fundamentals (*see* basics)
gain weight, 24, 34, 44, 197, 213, 223, 243, 279, 314, 316-317
genetics 22, 24, 136, 206, 209-210

glucose 39, 220, 224, 226
glycogen 29, 31-32, 39, 41-42, 44-46, 275
goals 11, 19, 45, 48, 66, 85, 89, 91-93, 95-99, 101-104, 106-107, 114, 116-117, 122-123, 128, 141, 146-147, 154-156, 161, 166, 178, 205-206, 216, 222, 257, 259, 308, 310-313, 315, 317-319
Gymnema Sylvestre 278
health 11, 14- 20, 33, 48, 63-65, 70, 81, 85, 95, 100, 108, 111, 113, 116, 119, 123-124, 126-127, 132, 134-137, 141, 144, 154, 159, 164, 169, 171, 176, 182-185, 202, 205, 220-221, 246, 257, 264, 272, 276-278, 285, 319, 321
heart rate 25, 124, 147, 149, 178, 181, 196, 220, 248
herbal stimulants 194
high-calorie diet 23, 213
high-rep 193, 216, 243
home gym 124
hunger 31, 33, 36, 154, 195, 286
immune system 25, 43, 201, 256
impulse decision, 165
impulse eating 72
injuries 48, 242-243, 248-250, 253
instant gratification 11, 125, 153-154, 160
intermediate exerciser 41, 45, 173, 188, 212, 218, 221-222, 233, 243, 306, 311
internal motivation 14, 18, 126
interval sprints, interval training 150, 159-160, 181

joints 188, 192, 243, 248-249, 254
junk food, 17, 61, 71-75, 79, 120, 161, 164-165, 244, 267, 272
Lean Rewards 117
lean tissue, lean body mass (*see also* muscle) 25, 29, 31-32, 35-36, 51, 58, 63-64, 161, 205, 226, 236, 256, 310
lose weight 14, 23-24, 26-27, 39, 44-45, 47, 49, 62, 96, 155, 178, 181-183, 195-196, 205, 216, 225, 279, 310, 311, 314, 319
low back 60, 133, 292, 296, 300-301, 303, 305
low-calorie 23, 25, 263, 268, 279, 288
low-calorie diet 23
low-carb 24, 39, 45-47, 57, 225, 265, 267, 270, 287
lower body 50, 52, 179, 202, 220, 278, 314
low-fat 42, 225, 263, 267-270, 284, 287
low-rep 193, 212, 243
lunges 51, 192, 201, 295
macronutrients 42, 155, 268
magazines 17, 129, 135-137, 141
maintenance 24, 26, 82, 220, 310
males, 25, 51, 53, 56, 135-136, 180, 182-183, 197-198, 213-216, 282, 321
malnutrition 43, 195
meal-replacement 266
measurements 109, 139, 162, 190
mesomorphs 316-317

metabolic rate 22, 28, 49, 181, 223, 317
metabolism, 21- 24, 28, 31-38, 40, 45, 47-50, 62-66, 89, 96, 175, 178-180, 194-197, 202, 205, 212, 214, 220-221, 223-224, 226-227, 256, 274, 279, 281, 289, 313-314, 323
micronnutrients (vitamins and minerals), 55, 62-64, 89, 120, 195, 257, 266, 271, 285
mind-to-muscle connection 149, 151
minerals (*see* micronutrients)
mission statement 77
moderation 12, 272
morbidly obese 196
motivation 16, 31, 70, 73, 89, 102-103, 106, 117, 120, 126-127, 245
muscle (*see also* lean tissue) 12, 22-25, 28-29, 31, 34-45, 47-48, 62-65, 91, 95, 135-137, 141-142, 147, 149, 151, 155, 158, 161, 169, 178-182, 188-190, 192-194, 196-197, 200-203, 205-206, 208-210, 212-214, 216, 225-227, 234, 236, 238, 241, 243, 248-249, 251, 253-255, 268, 275-276, 281, 289, 292, 300, 306, 310-312, 314-317, 319, 321, 323
muscular failure, 50, 149-151, 173, 193, 212, 234, 241
negative thinking 89
negatives 212
nutrient partitioning 47-48

nutrition 14, 42-43, 45-47, 63, 95, 111, 113-114, 117, 119, 128-129, 135, 137-139, 141, 147, 151, 155, 169, 206, 225, 257, 265-268, 272, 276-277, 279, 320-321
obesity 114, 183
orthopedic 199, 250
orthotics 133
osteoporosis 64, 114, 198
overeating 30, 34, 37, 40, 42, 79, 152, 156, 165, 222, 281, 317
overreaching 254
overtraining 48, 223, 242, 253-254, 312
patience 15, 17, 34
planning 14, 46, 75, 125, 146-147, 174, 202, 239, 272
points system 119-121, 125, 161
positive obsession 11, 122-123, 128
positive self-talk 11, 86-88
post-exercise calorie burn 49, 160, 222
post-workout 181, 265-266
priorities 84, 114, 123, 124, 136, 192, 223, 319
procrastination 81, 83
progressive resistance training 23, 235
prohormones (*see* andro)
pronation 132
protein 23, 39, 45, 66, 136, 155, 196, 201, 263-266, 268-270, 283, 285, 317
psychology 14, 71, 138
push-up 173-174, 296-297
recovery (*see also* rest) 45, 63, 150, 158, 160, 201-202, 221, 242, 253-257, 265

recreation (*see* sports)
repetition, rep 52, 123, 136, 149, 174, 192, 212, 233, 243, 291, 293, 311, 313, 316-318
resistance training 22, 28-31, 39, 45, 67, 100, 114, 116-117, 120, 124, 136, 141, 149, 150-151, 159, 174, 176, 178-182, 189, 192, 201, 203, 205, 212, 214-216, 218, 220, 224-228, 233-234, 236, 243-244, 246, 248-249, 253, 257, 265, 268, 310-311, 315-317, 319
rest 12, 16, 33, 55, 57, 59, 65, 72, 81-82, 85, 119, 147, 149-150, 154, 174, 188, 192, 199-203, 206, 233, 236, 241, 244-245, 249-250, 252-257, 268, 272-273, 306-307, 309-311, 313, 315-318
restaurant 74-75, 186, 283-287
reward 18, 34, 82, 104, 116-117, 119, 120, 125, 154, 161
rock-bottom 70
saccharin 277, 278
safety 192
scale 29, 30, 34, 36, 120, 161, 163, 166, 179, 275
self-sabotage 33
serotonin 279
set point 37, 206
shoes, sneakers 91, 132-133, 193
short-term pleasure 17, 70, 164
side crunch 304
skipping meals 41, 66
sleep 65-66, 89, 93, 199, 202, 253, 256-257, 313, 315, 317-318, 323
slips 75

sneakers (*see* shoes)
split routine 201, 233
sports, recreation 61, 235
sports drink 39, 193
squat 193, 208, 292-294, 306
starvation 25, 41
steady-pace cardio 48-49
stevia 278
stress 81, 82, 202
stretching 248-251
stubborn fat 183, 215
success, 1, 3, 11, 18, 41, 86-87, 90, 93-95, 100, 103, 105, 107, 120-121, 123, 128, 145-146, 153-154, 168-169, 171, 205, 236, 255, 259
sucralose 278
sugar 11, 22, 33, 44, 46-47, 53-54, 57-58, 71, 120, 130, 132, 264, 267-268, 276-279, 284-285, 288
supersets 234, 313, 315, 317
supination 132
supplements 20, 32, 62-64, 116, 135-136, 155, 160, 193-194, 197, 199, 220, 268, 277, 312
survival (perceived threat to),
survival mechanism 24-25, 32-34, 37, 41, 71-72
systems 25, 33, 35, 43, 125, 128, 195, 212, 244
testosterone 158, 197, 213-215, 281
The 80/20 Rule 12, 75, 77, 119, 195, 272-273, 275
thermogenics 193
time off (from exercise or dieting) 181, 221, 236, 241, 255, 313, 315, 317, 318

token 30, 40, 117, 119
toning 36, 44, 52-53, 66, 74, 98, 161, 205, 209, 268, 312
trainer (*see* fitness trainer)
trigger 72-73, 156, 159-160, 165
urge management tool 157, 163, 166-167
visualization 91, 93
vitamins (*see* micronutrients)
warm-up 147
water 29-32, 36, 45, 62, 91, 95, 109, 162, 193, 234, 263-264, 268-269, 275, 279, 285
water weight 29-31, 95, 275
weight loss 1, 3, 16-18, 23, 25-26, 29, 32-33, 38-39, 45-46, 49, 53, 62, 64, 66, 95-96, 116, 180-182, 195, 202, 209, 213, 220-222, 225, 244, 268, 273-274, 281, 287, 315
willpower 15, 33-34, 71-72
workout 17, 19, 38-41, 45-46, 48-49, 79, 82, 84-85, 87, 91, 93, 100, 116-117, 119-121, 126, 131-133, 135, 137, 139, 147, 149-150, 158, 161-162, 173-176, 178, 180-181, 183, 185-186, 192-193, 199, 201-203, 216, 221-223, 226, 233-235, 238-239, 242, 244, 248, 251, 253-255, 257, 265-266, 270, 274, 289, 298, 303, 306-309, 313, 315, 317-319, 321
youthful 22, 37
yo-yo dieting 31, 34, 213